C000181224

OPIUM

A JOURNEY THROUGH TIME

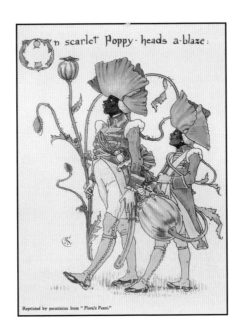

n scarlet Poppy-heads a-blaze:

Reprinted by permission from "Flora's Feast."

Title page: Illustration from 'Flora's Feast' by Walter Crane.

Published in 2004 by Mercury Books
20 Bloomsbury Street
London WC1B 3JH

© 2004 Mercury Books

Designed and produced for Mercury Books
by Open Door Limited, Langham, Rutland

Edited by Stephen Chumbley

All rights reserved. No part of this publication may be reproduced
or transmitted in any form or by any means, electronic or
mechanical, including photocopying, recording or any information
storage and retrieval system, without prior permission in writing
from the copyright owner.

Title: Opium, A Journey Through Time
ISBN: 1-904668-50-X

OPIUM

A JOURNEY THROUGH TIME

COLIN R. SHEARING

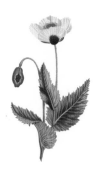

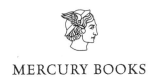

MERCURY BOOKS

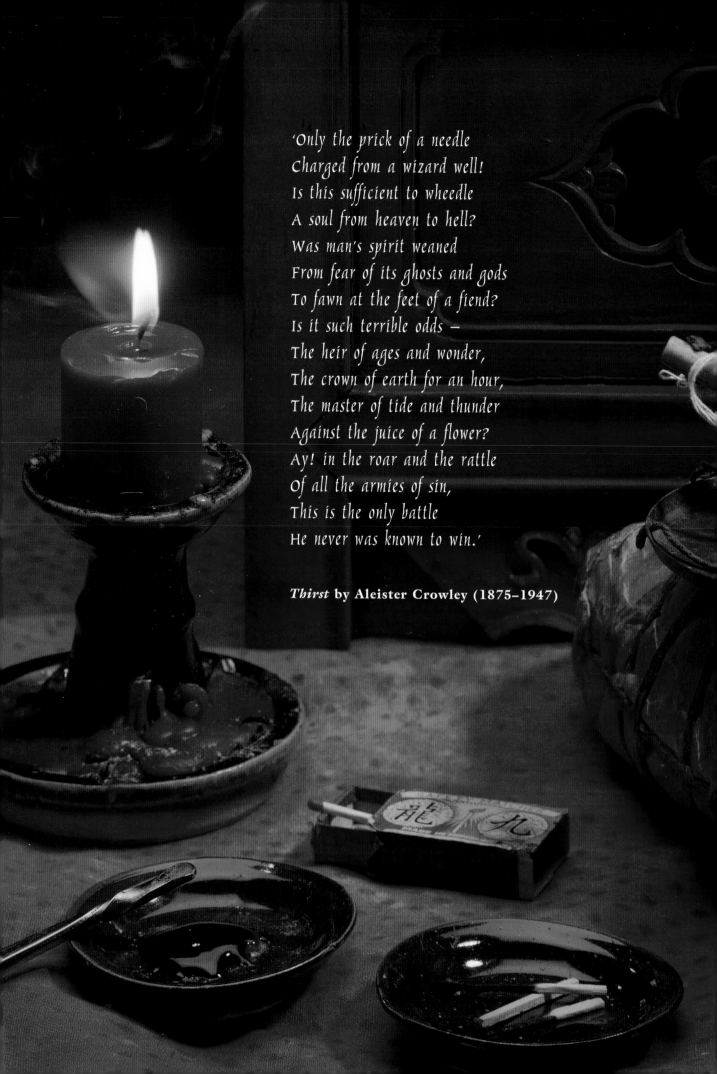

'Only the prick of a needle
Charged from a wizard well!
Is this sufficient to wheedle
A soul from heaven to hell?
Was man's spirit weaned
From fear of its ghosts and gods
To fawn at the feet of a fiend?
Is it such terrible odds –
The heir of ages and wonder,
The crown of earth for an hour,
The master of tide and thunder
Against the juice of a flower?
Ay! in the roar and the rattle
Of all the armies of sin,
This is the only battle
He never was known to win.'

Thirst by Aleister Crowley (1875–1947)

CONTENTS

Opium is one of the most evocative words in the English language. It is derived from the ancient Greek word for the sap of the poppy pod ('opion') but in its long history it has changed from being seen as a gift from the gods to the scourge of modern society and yet paradoxically both statements are true. Huge fortunes have been spent on both cultivating it and attempting to destroy it, but still it remains and it seems impossible to imagine a world without it. After all, it is simply a flower, like many others, and yet it conjures to us all powerful, exotic images of seedy opium dens, with Fu Manchu-like fiends lurking in smoke-filled brothels, dirty hypodermic needles left in public lavatories, AIDS sufferers, hopeless addicts lying in squalor, ruthless drug barons and gangsters for whom opium is a means to great wealth for a small capital outlay. Poisoners kill with it and have done so for thousands of

Refined opium being spooned into china ramekins. Each ramekin contains enough opium for two or three smokes.

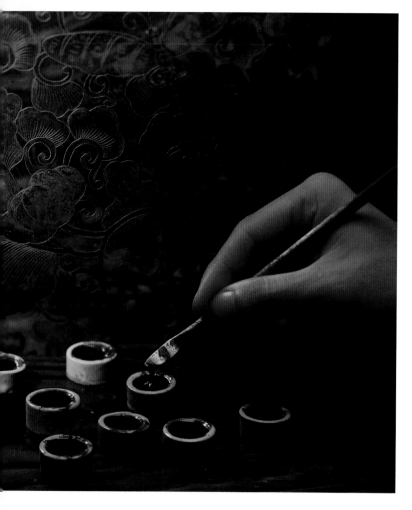

years, terrorists are financed by it, urban crime seems fuelled by it and arms dealers use it as their currency. Opium and its derivatives account for an illicit multinational trade which is larger than the gross economies of some countries. To the addict, opium and its derivatives are the stuff of dreams, an escape from reality and a temporary entry into paradise followed by a rapid descent into hell.

In short, society seems undermined by opium yet, for all this, opium has its benign side. For the terminal patient opium and its derivatives, heroin and morphine, bring a blessed relief from the indignities of pain and suffering; for them it is an angel of mercy. Many an

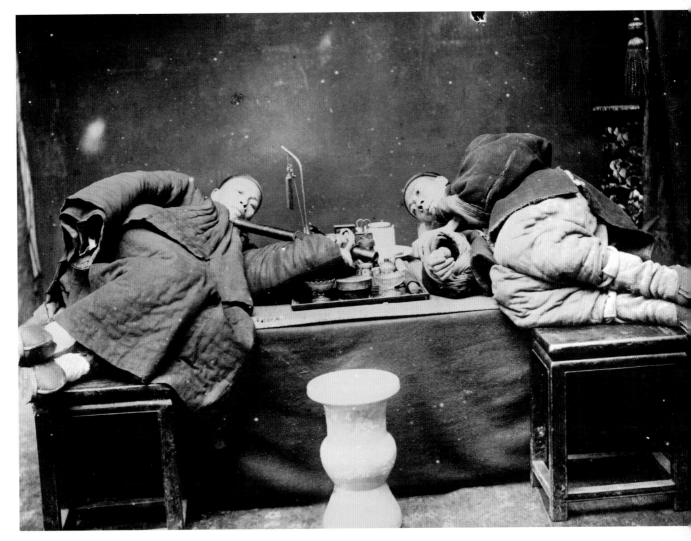

artist has been fuelled by its muse-like qualities and some of our most prominent literary, musical and artistic figures could not have managed without the inspiration it brought to their work.

Two men share a pipe in a Chinese opium den.

How can such a small, fragile flower be responsible for both relieving and causing so much suffering to humanity? To try and address this question this book will be investigating that complex relationship. Opium and its derivatives are, it seems, all things to all men and have been for thousands of years. The story goes back 5,000 years or more and has its origins in the beginnings of human society and there seems little doubt that opium will be there to help relieve the suffering when civilisation itself comes to an end.

*'It is difficult to live without opium after having known it
because it is difficult, after knowing opium, to take earth
seriously. And unless one is a saint, it is difficult to live
without taking earth seriously.'*

Jean Cocteau (1889–1963)

There are various theories as to how and where the opium poppy, papaver somniferum Linnaeus, originated. The opium poppy was taxonomically classified by Linnaeus, the pioneering founder of botany, in 1753 as papaver somniferum, 'papaver' being its genus and 'somniferum' referring to its 'sleep inducing' properties from the Latin word 'somnus'. There are a number of plants belonging to the poppy family Papaveraceae but the opium poppy is the only type of poppy of the many strains that contains commercially viable amounts of opium. It is believed to have evolved through centuries of breeding and cultivation from the wild strain Papaver setigerum.

Before 4000 BC, the opium poppy was being cultivated in the Tigris/Euphrates river systems of Lower Mesopotamia. The earliest reference was mentioned in a Sumerian text dated 4000 BC. The ancient Sumerians called it 'hul gil' meaning the plant of joy. The Sumerians, the world's earliest known civilisation and agriculturalists, used it for medicinal purposes and quite possibly in their religious ceremonies. It seems therefore that the Sumerians not only gave humankind literacy, but one of its greatest medicines and also one of its greatest problems. At a cave burial site in Albunol, near Grenada in Southern Spain, the Neolithic site called Cueva de Los Murcielagos (the Cave of the Milky Way), capsules of opium poppy were discovered in woven grass bags around the bodies. It appears that opium may have been included in their funerary rites and rituals. In the early Bronze Age (1600 BC), poppy seed mixture cakes were found in Swiss Foreland. This area between the Alps and the Jura Mountains may have been part of a trade route from the Rhine, although the Rivers Danube, Rhone and Po also converge there. From Switzerland, the route of opium then spreads to the Eastern Mediterranean and Northern Europe.

By the end of the second millennium BC, knowledge of opium was widespread throughout Europe, the Middle East and North Africa. The Sumerian invention of writing spread gradually to other societies and cultures, to the Assyrians and the Babylonians, and it is from this knowledge that the Egyptians probably learnt the skill of cultivation. In sources such as the *Veterinary, Gynaecological* and *Therapeutic papyri* references of opium are included in some 700 remedies. The *Veterinary* and the *Gynaecological papyri* date from 1850–1700 BC and were both found in Kahun, now known as Lahun. The former was written in Egyptian hieroglyphs, in a script reserved for sacred texts and the latter was so overused by its ancient owner that it was found to have been repaired with a patch.

The *Therapeutic papyrus* of Thebes dates back to the sixteenth century BC, and is also known as the *Papyrus of Ebers* after the Egyptologist who discovered it Georg Moritz Ebers (1837–98). Within its hieroglyphs are contained the diagnosis and treatments for numerous ailments such as asthma, headaches and digestive disorders. Some 700 of the 877 prescriptions involve opium, amongst more unusual ingredients of their Materia Medica such as bile and hippopotamus fat. It has a section which details opium as a remedy to calm restless children from colic, a practice which was to continue until the first half of the twentieth century. However, the earlier prescription, rather than being an opiate/camphor tincture, demanded that the opium be mixed with fly droppings, pulped, sieved and taken for four days instead.

Cuts on the pods of *opium poppies ooze white latex – the gum that produces opium. Incisions are made daily and the gum harvested. This continues until the pods are exhausted.*

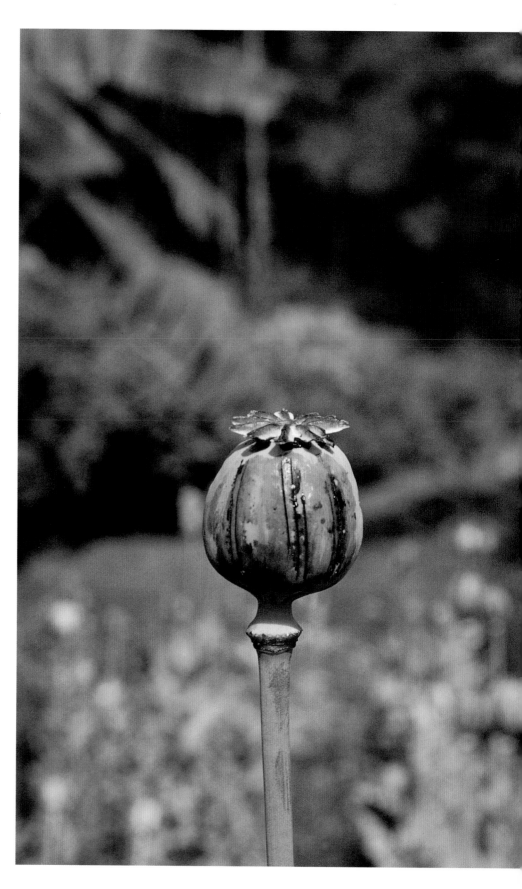

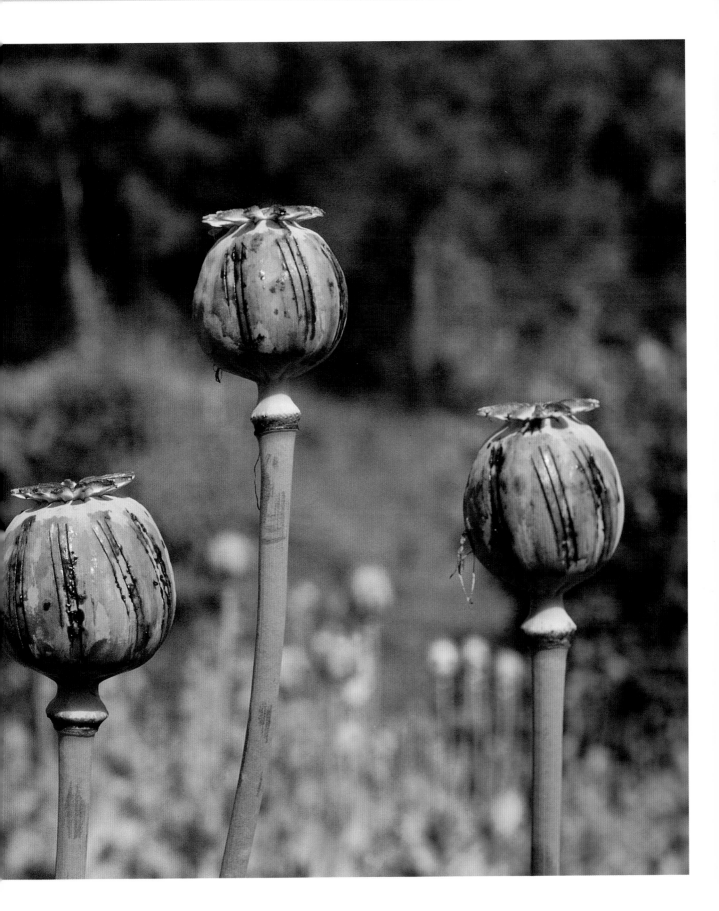

The earliest Egyptian find of opium itself comes from a sample which was discovered in the tomb of Cha, dating to the fifteenth century BC. The Egyptian poppy fields became legendary and under the rule of Thutmose IV, Akhenaten and most famously King Tutankhamun, the opium trade flourished. In Thebes, on the Nile, the Egyptians used to cultivate opium and called the preparation 'thebacium'. In the thirteenth century BC the Egyptians were known to trade opium via the Mediterranean Sea into Europe and Greece. Poppy juice is also mentioned in seventh-century BC Assyrian medical tablets contained in the Royal Library of the Babylonian King Asurbanipal, although these are believed to be copies of earlier texts. Doctors at this time considered opium a cure for almost every ailment, sometimes mixing it with liquorice or balsam: of 115 herbal or vegetable concoctions mentioned in the text, 42 concern opium, which was collected early in the morning by women and children who scraped the congealed sap off wounds made in the poppies with a small iron scoop. For the Greek civilisation opium was a commonplace herbal derivative. The word for poppy was 'mekon'. In the third century BC, Theophrastus referred to the sap of the poppy as 'opion' while he called poppy juice 'meconion' (obtained by pressing the entire plant). This suggests that he had a specific knowledge that the sap contained a substance and that he may have been acquainted with separating it out, although at the time, the general method of taking opium was to crush the pod in wine and steep it in a honey and water solution. The word 'meconium', used as a medical term for the faecal matter of a newborn baby, takes its etymology from mekon, due to its similar appearance to the sap.

The method of incising a poppy to gather the sap was developed by the Assyrians and is used to this day. The technique was lost but was reinvented or rediscovered about AD 40 by Scribonius Largus, physician to the Emperor Claudius. Theophrastus, while noting that opium induced sleep and numbed pain did, not consider its effects upon the brain which were generally disregarded, although the philosopher Diagoras 'the Atheist' of Melos, living in the third century BC, was aware of the drug's snare. He declared it was better to suffer pain than to become dependent on opium.

Apart from its medicinal use, opium also served the Greeks in a spiritual or occult capacity, being employed by initiates to the cult of Demeter. The medical priests of Aesculapeius administered opium to those who visited their sanctuary at Epidaurus. Clients would sleep inside the temple whilst the priests procured healing dreams for them. As long as opium was in the hands of priests, it was regarded as a metaphysical substance. This supernatural attitude, however, was dismissed by Hippocrates (460–357 BC). Considered the father of modern medicine, he disassociated himself from the magical attributes of opium but instead mentioned that it was useful as a cathartic, hypnotic, narcotic and stiptic. He suggested drinking hypnotic meconion mixed with nettle seeds to cure leucorrhea (vaginal discharge) and uterine suffocation. Hippocrates was of the opinion that it should be used sparingly and under control, a stipulation which exists to this day in the Hippocratic oath which states 'I will neither give a deadly drug to anybody who asks for it, nor will I make a suggestion to this effect'.

In its early history, opium was not seen in the same way as it is today. It was considered a gift from the gods, its medicinal properties were valued and for most people it was for this reason alone that the plant was so revered. In fact, the main social addiction issue in Ancient Greece was not opium, but alcohol. A vast proportion of opium use would remain confined and passive, whereas in contrast, alcohol, and wine in particular, would be the fuel for many disturbances. Ironically, this parallels today's world. The Greeks had laws concerning alcohol consumption in much the same way that modern society does, age being the major factor. Experience, being an attribute that was valued more than anything else, caused Plato to write in his Laws that 'Wine had been granted to elders by the gods as a potion to lighten the sourness of old age'. The word narcotic comes from the Greek word 'Narkosis' for benumbing/deadening. From medicine to philosophy it was not long before opium began to appear in stories.

In Homer's epic tale *The Odyssey*, which is about the travels of Odysseus, he mentions 'Nepenthe', the drink of forgetfulness, which is reputedly made from an Egyptian opium formula. When Telemachus visits King Menelaus and his wife Helen in Sparta, a wedding banquet is to be held but all the guests are grieving for the loss of Odysseus and his comrades during the Trojan War. In order to lighten everyone's spirits, Helen prepares a special draught

'Then Helen, daughter of Zeus, turned to new thoughts. Presently she cast a drug into the wine whereof they drank, a drug to lull all pain and anger, and bring forgetfulness of every sorrow. Whoso should drink a draught thereof, when it is mingled in the bowl, on that day he would let no tear fall down his cheeks, not though his mother and his father died, not though men slew his brother or dear son with the sword before his face, and his own eyes beheld it. Medicines of such virtue and so helpful had the daughter of Zeus, which Polydamna, the wife of Thoen, had given her, a woman of Egypt, where earth the grain-giver yields herbs in greatest plenty, many that are healing in the cup, and many baneful'.

Homer (1000 BC)

In the Bible, it is clear that the medical knowledge of the Egyptians was shared by Moses, as he had grown up in the Egyptian royal family. This knowledge would have included opium. In Book 44, Acts 7, Verse 22 of the Old Testament it states 'And Moses was learned in all the wisdom of the Egyptians and was mighty in words and in deeds'.

A solution of opium in alcohol was used by the Greeks as a tranquilliser to banish fear and anguish. It might also have been used to promote 'Dutch courage' in warriors going into battle. When the Greek civilisation was usurped by the Empire of Rome, more than works of art and treasures were plundered and brought to Italy. Literature which included philosophy and medicine were brought and an essential part of the Materia Medica learnt on the battlefields of foreign campaigns included the painkilling properties of opium.

Galen, the last of the great Greek physicians and the author of some five hundred texts, enthused that opium was 'a glorious panacea', that resisted poison. It was also beneficial in the healing of 'venomous bites, cured headaches, vertigo, deafness, epilepsy, apoplexy, poor sight, bronchitis, asthma, coughs, the spitting of blood, colic, jaundice, hardening of the spleen, kidney stones, urinary complaints, fever, dropsy, leprosy, menstrual problems, melancholy and all other pestilences'. He also popularised the use of one of the early opium concoctions named 'Mithridate'. He advocated it to all his patients including Marcus Aurelius, and the Emperors Commodus and Severus. He studied and published his findings on the toxic effects of opium and even at this early date understood the concept of tolerance, being the ability of the body to withstand larger and larger successive doses, which requires increasing the dose to gain the same effect as time goes on.

Virgil also mentions opium in his works; in both the *Aeneid* and the *Georgics*. He calls it a soporific. His lines 'spargens humida melle soperiferumque paparva' ('giving dewy honey and soporific poppies') and 'Lethaeo perfusa papavera somno' ('poppies soaked with the sleep of

Lethe') from the First Book of the Georgics indicate very clearly the accepted capabilities of the drug. The Roman writer and natural historian Pliny the Elder, who lived in the first century AD, wrote much about the Materia Medica of his time and culture. He observed that poppy seed was a useful hypnotic, whilst the poppy latex was effective in treating headaches, arthritis and healing wounds but warned that 'taken in too large quantities is productive of sleep unto death even'. To the Romans, opium was not only a painkiller or religious drug but was a useful poison and for suicide it was a gentle release into death. The Carthaginian Hannibal ended his life with it in 183 BC to avoid capture by the Romans. Opium was the ideal assassin's tool as it was easily found and easily disguised in food or wine. It induced a seemingly innocent death as if in sleep. In one such instance in 367 BC the son of Dionysus (the Tyrant of Syracuse) made an arrangement with the court doctors for his father to overdose on it and in AD 55 Agrippina, the Emperor Claudius's last wife, poisoned her 14-year-old stepson Britannicus with opium so that her own son, Nero, would inherit the throne. For leisure use, opium was eaten mixed with honey to suppress its bitterness. The eating of opium increased as the knowledge of its beneficial properties became more widely known. In the second century AD, it was stated in the *Sextus Empericus* that Lysis could take four drachms of poppy juice without being incapacitated. To be so tolerant of the drug suggests that he was a well-established user as such a quantity would have killed a first-time user.

In Rome we start to see opium becoming more or less the ancient equivalent to aspirin. The potent ability of the plant to ease everyday ailments made it popular amongst the citizens of Rome and its power to considerably alleviate pain made it popular on the battlefield. Indeed, the poppy was so well known that in later years of the Empire it was found on Roman coinage and there are also friezes depicting the poppy in the

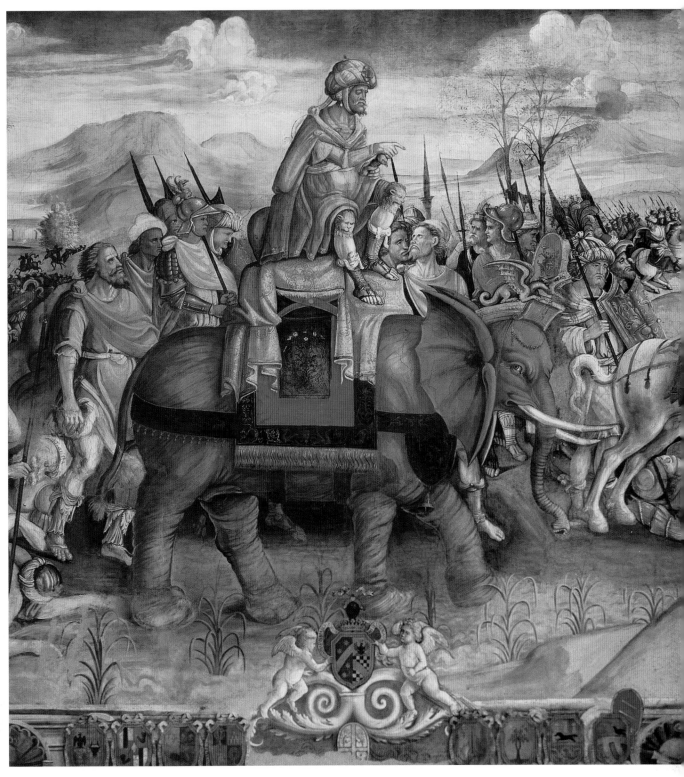

remains of Pompeii (the disaster in which Pliny the Elder was to die). However, by the seventh century AD opium had largely fallen into disuse for medicinal purposes within the Greek culture.

Detail of 'Hannibal in Italy' attributed to Jocopo Ripanda.

Curiously neither the Romans nor the Greeks regarded opium as an international trading commodity. However, the Arabs did: they had used opium as a painkiller for centuries, having translated many of the Greek texts and it was they who developed and organised the production of and trading in opium which has existed ever since. After the death of Mohammed, the Prophet, in AD 632, the Arab Empire rapidly expanded due to his successors, the four Khalifs, who sought to spread the faith of Islam throughout southern Europe and North Africa, and opium was the perfect trading commodity for them. At this time however, it was only used as a medicine, except in India where it was regarded as a form of recreation as well. Islamic traders introduced opium into China during the eighth century Tang Dynasty and, by the ninth century Arab scholars were publishing texts on 'Af-yum' as opium was known. The knowledge was spread by Arab merchants and physicians and the study of opium at this time reached its height in the person of the Islamic philosopher, Abu Ali al Husein Abdallah ibn Sina, know by his Latin name Avicenna in the medieval world. Ibn Sina was born in 980 and spent most of his life in Persia, living in a palace in Isfahan, a place noted for its opium production. His interests included mathematics, medicine and poetry. He had the privilege of his own harem and although the Koran taught that alcohol was forbidden, Ibn Sina was known to praise the virtues of both wine and poppies in his poetry. He wrote over 400 books in his lifetime and his most famous in the Western world was the *Canon of Medicine*, a five-volume book that brought Greek, Arab, Persian, Indian as well as his own personal knowledge of medicine together. It was translated into Latin by Christian scholars in the twelfth century and was used as the standard for monastic medical knowledge thereafter. Ironically Avicenna died in 1037 from what was believed to be an accidental overdose of opium mixed with wine.

In Europe, the use of opium had declined in line with the Roman Empire. Opium then re-appeared at the time of the Crusades as the Christian knights learnt about it from the Arab warriors that they fought in the Holy Land. Once again opium stopped being purely a medicine and became a substance of legend. In Europe, the returning knights would recount tales of exotic lands which would become the Chronicles of the Crusades. One of the most popular stories was that of 'The Old Man of the Mountains', or Hasan Al Sabbah, who was the leader of a group of holy warriors, the Assassins (from which our modern day word is derived). He created a garden of earthly paradise for his followers who spent their days enraptured by the powers of magical herbs, with fountains of milk and honey, set amongst green lawns and attended by dancing houris dressed in silk and gold. This story of his forbidden garden joined itself to older myths and became an image lurking below the consciousness of European literature. The legend of the Old Man of the Mountains with his young assassins and the drugs he gave them, was caught up by Marco Polo, Mandeville and Purchas and they brought it to the poetic imagination of Europe.

European writers began to be influenced by opium. In Chaucer's *Canterbury Tales*, in the prologue of the Doctor's Tale, Chaucer tells that the Doctor was well read on Aesculapeius, Hippocrates, Dioscorides, Galen, and Avicenna, who were all noted for expounding the virtues of opium. He based his character the 'Doctor of Physick' on John of Gaddesden (1280–1361), a doctor who studied at Merton College, Oxford and whose manuscript, the *Rosa Medicinae* also mentions opium.

After the Moors were driven out from Spain by Ferdinand and Isabella in the fifteenth century, the influence of the Islamic traders diminished and so opium was next taken up as a trading commodity by the Venetians. Venice was an ideal port in terms of its location, and it acted as a sea-faring bridge between the East and West. Opium was imported to Venice from the Middle East along with spices, and when Columbus sailed to discover the New World it was one of the commodities he was instructed to bring back, as were the explorers Cabot, Magellan and Vasco da Gama.

It was the influence of the Knights Templar that we see here, as all these mariners sailed under the cross of the Knights Templar who were, along with the Knights Hospitaller, renowned for their proficiency in medicine, largely learnt from their interactions with the Arab world during the Crusades.

In the thirteenth century two monks by the names of Hugo of Lucca and his successor Theoderic of Bologna experimented with opium to ease pain during spinal surgery. They rediscovered what was termed a 'spongia somnifera'. As the name implies, this was a sponge soaked with opium and other substances such as henbane which was held over the patient's nose and acted as an anaesthetic. This technique had also been used by the Romans and is even referred to in the Crucifixion. In England and across much of north-western Europe opium was medicinally employed, mainly for its narcotic properties. John Arderne (1307– 90), a renowned surgeon, used salves and potions containing opium to procure sleep and also applied it externally as a crude anaesthetic during surgery. Opium was the essential ingredient of the some of the mainstays of the medieval apothecary, particularly theriacs (treaclelike antidotes) such as Mithridatum, Philonium and Diascordium. These were common paliatives and general antidotes to a vast range of medical conditions. This use continued with opium seemingly being a gift from God although some of the monasteries did not approve of anything that reduced pain, believing this to be God's will to suffer.

Another opium-based substance was 'Laudanum', first developed by Paracelsus (1490–1541). He studied and taught medicine at the University of Basle, usually in German rather than Latin, and was taught alchemy by the Bishop of Würzburg. Paracelsus's approach to medicine was revolutionary. He launched attacks against Avicenna's *Canon of Medicine* by burning it publicly and in doing so dismissed Galen's Humoral theory of disease. He heavily criticised physicians, apothecaries and surgeons for

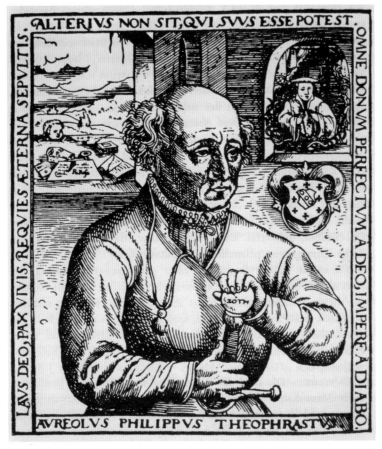

ALTERIVS NON SIT, QVI SVVS ESSE POTEST.

LAVS DEO, PAX VIVIS, REQVIES ÆTERNA SEPVLTIS.

OMNE DONVM PERFECTVM A DEO, IMPERFECTVM A DIABO.

AVREOLVS PHILIPPVS THEOPHRASTVS

Engraved portrait of Paracelsus from his book, 'Astronomica et Astrologica Pouscula'.

duping the public with cures that did not work or practising in ways that were potentially lethal. He travelled around Europe and the Islamic countries, interrogating ordinary people in his belief that practical knowledge far outweighed that of scholars, thus flying in the face of the establishment. He was rumoured to carry the 'Elixir of Life' in the pommel of his double-handed sword. Unlike many, Paracelsus believed that medicine rather than gold was the true call of the alchemist and referred to opium as the 'Stone of Immortality' which was also another name given to the Holy Grail of earlier legends. He wrote 'I possess a secret remedy which I call 'Laudanum' and which is superior to all other heroic remedies'. The ingredients he used were 25% opium, mixed with henbane, crushed pearls and coral, amber, musk, and cryptically bezoar stone, the bone from the heart of a stag and finally powdered unicorn's horn! Paracelsus's success and reputation amongst the ordinary people did much to advance opium use. It was Paracelsus who paved the way for modern medicine by taking it out of the hands of scholars and putting it into the hands of the people.

Following in Paracelsus's footsteps was Nicholas Culpeper. He studied at Cambridge University although he did not complete his studies. He became incensed at physicians who charged vast amounts for toxic concoctions and criticised their practices of bloodletting. Instead he preferred to go out into the field and find cures available in the immediate surroundings. He wrote a number of books including *The English Midwife* and in 1652 published his book *The English Physitian* better known as *Culpeper's Complete Herbal*, which gave him the modern-day title of founder of alternative medicine.

> 'The Herb is Lunar, and of the juyce of it is made Opium, onely for lucre of money they cheat you, and tell you it is a kinde of Tear, or some such like thing that drops from Poppies when they weep, and that is some where beyond the Sea, I know not where, beyond the Moon.'

Nicholas Culpeper (1616–54)

Thomas Sydenham, who was nicknamed the English Hippocrates, was one of the leading English physicians of the seventeenth century. He trained at Oxford and in 1666 he invented his own liquid laudanum. He used the name 'laudanum' that had been coined by Paracelsus (from the latin verb 'laudare', meaning 'to praise'). Laudanum became a common opium preparation; it was a tincture usually made with sherry wine and spices such as saffron, cinnamon and cloves to disguise the bitterness. The combination of alcohol and opium was seen as the most normal and convenient way for Westerners to partake of the poppy for a number of centuries, even though it could potentially kill.

'Its merit consists in being of a more convenient form, and more uniform in the action of its doses. It can be given with wine, distilled water, or any other liquid. And here I cannot but break out in praise of the great God, the Giver of all good things who hath granted to the human race, as a comfort in their afflictions, no medicine of the value of opium, either in regard to the number of diseases that is can control, or its efficiency in extirpating them. As all forms of opium come alike from the poppy, it is an attempt upon our credulity to pretend that the viruses of narcotics in general, and of opium in particular, are due to any artificial or peculiar process on the part of the preparer. Whoever will be guided by experience, and will diligently and frequently compare the effects of the natural juice with the effect of its artificial preparations, will discover that there is no difference between them; and will be well assured that the wonderful effects of the remedy are the effects of its own natural virtue and excellence, and are not due to any skill of any clever artifice whatever. So necessary an instrument is opium in the hand of a skilful man, that medicine would be a cripple without it; and whoever understands it well, will do more with it alone than he could well hope to do from any single medicine. To know it only as a means of procuring sleep, or of allaying pain, or of checking diarrhea is to know it only by halves. Like a Delphic sword, it can be used for many purposes besides. Of cordials it is the best that has hitherto been discovered in Nature'

Thomas Sydenham (1624–89)

One of Sydenham's pupils, Thomas Dover, developed his own product called Dover's Powder, which first appeared in the *London Pharmacopoeia* of 1788 and was still being used up until the Second World War. Thomas Dover, after studying under Sydenham became a privateer and commanded a vessel called *The Duke* with which he raided the coast of South America and on February 2nd 1709 he rescued Alexander Selkirk, the shipwrecked sailor who had spent 4 years and 4 months on the island of Juan Fernandez, and so became the prototype for Defoe's Robinson Crusoe. Dover's Powder was described as a diaphoretic, a substance to promote sweating and so allow a fever to run its course, and he gives the method of its preparation in his 1733 book *The Ancient Physician's Legacy to his Country. Being What he has collected himself in Forty-nine Years Practice: Or, An Account of the several Diseases incident to Mankind, described in so plain a Manner, that any Person may know the Nature of his own Disease*. In the book the original formula was 1oz each of opium, liquorice and ipecacuanha with 4oz each of saltpetre and vitriolated tartar to which Dover added that 'some apothecaries have desired their patients to make their wills before they venture upon so large a dose'. The off-the-shelf version was somewhat weaker, being made of 10 grains each of opium, ipecacuanha, and sulphate of potash.

As scientific studies increased a greater understanding of the properties of opium was achieved. Its occult connotations were gradually abandoned and concerns arose about its addictive nature. Doubts were expressed about its ability as a panacea. Doctor Samuel Johnson, the inventor of the first English dictionary, took opium on occasion, if only for medicinal purposes, as did his biographer James Boswell who used it to cure headaches and stomach trouble. In Boswell's *Life of Johnson* the biographer recorded on Sunday, March 23rd 1783: 'I breakfasted with Dr Johnson, who seemed much relieved having taken opium the night before. He however protested against it as a remedy that should be given with the utmost reluctance and only in extreme necessity. I mentioned how commonly it was used in Turkey, and that therefore, it could not be so pernicious as he apprehended. He grew warm and said, "Turks take opium and Christians take opium; but Russell, in his account of Aleppo, tells us that it is disgraceful in Turkey to take too much opium, as it is with us to get drunk. Sir, it is amazing how things are exaggerated".'

Dr. Johnson and Boswell in Fleet Street, London.

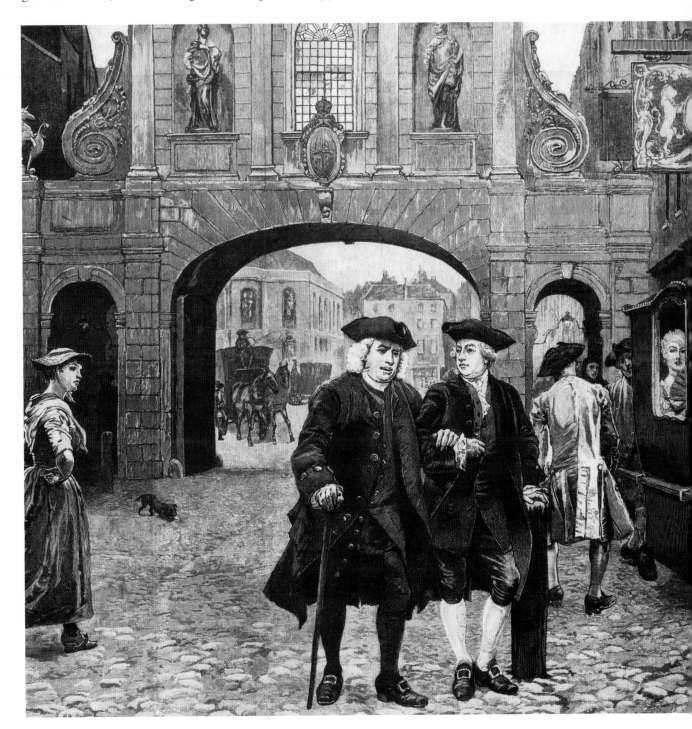

During the late fifteenth century, Arab traders had already helped spread the popularity of opium through southern Europe, north Africa, India and China. Although the usual trade routes were slow, there were many explorers who were eager to find a way of sourcing goods like opium, spices, herbs and tea without having to rely on middlemen. Vasco da Gama, the Portuguese explorer, managed to set up a trade monopoly with India until 1600. Over the next 200 years various countries challenged Portugal's exclusivity over the opium market. Eventually England was granted a concession on opium trading by the Indian ruling body. The Portuguese had also set up a monopoly with the Chinese in 1557 which was dissolved in 1685, allowing the British to set up trade from Canton by 1715. A major player in this was the East India Company which was formed by 218 Knights and Merchants of the City of London and granted its Royal Charter on December 31st 1600.

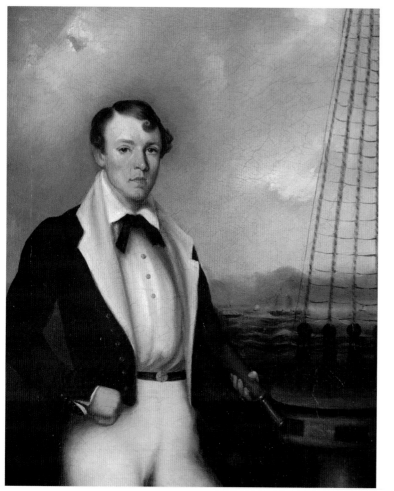

The portrait of an English midshipman relaxing after a gruelling voyage from Calcutta.

The East India Company initially made little impact on the Dutch-controlled spice trade at the time, but eventually went on to establish serious military dominance and an influential political empire for Britain in the East. Up until the late Elizabethan age the English were regarded by the then-dominant European powers of Spain and France as uncultured, barbaric and less advanced than their European neighbours. Because Dutch trading was so strong, the East India Company had to take what it could, often resulting in piracy and underhand deals. It is thought that the swashbuckling pirate role that the

East India Company played appealed to the romantic character of the fourth Moghul Emperor Jehangir who made Captain William Hawkins commander of his cavalry. Within 200 years the Moghul Empire itself would be in the hands of 'John Company', as the East India Company was affectionately known. By the middle of the seventeenth century the East India Company was trading alongside Arab and Indian merchants in the East, shipping goods including cloth from southern India to Sumatra, and coffee from Arabia to India. Gradually, as they built up their power base in India, they opened up trading posts in Madras and Calcutta. After creating these secure foundations the Company was able to seek out new markets and sources for trading products. Although the Company had failed to set up a stable trading post in Japan, they were amongst the first to penetrate China.

A British tea clipper under full sail – speed was the key to a good profit. The first tea to arrive in London each year commanded the highest prices.

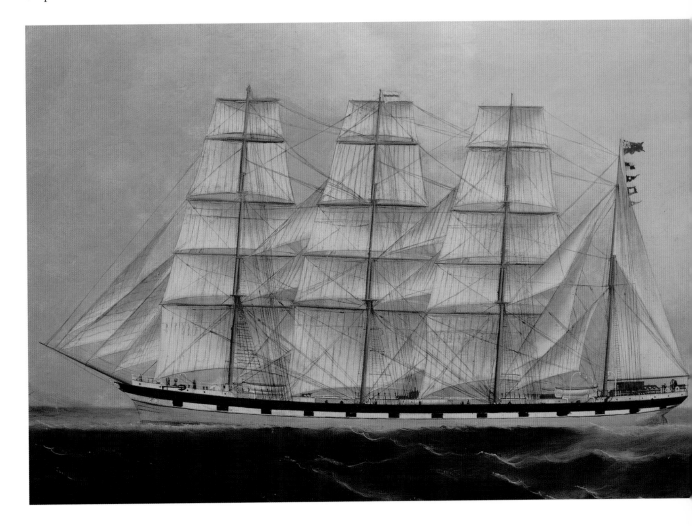

Canton Harbour c.1840. Visible in the background are the flags of four non-Chinese trading companies on the warehouses built just outside the western area of Canton city.

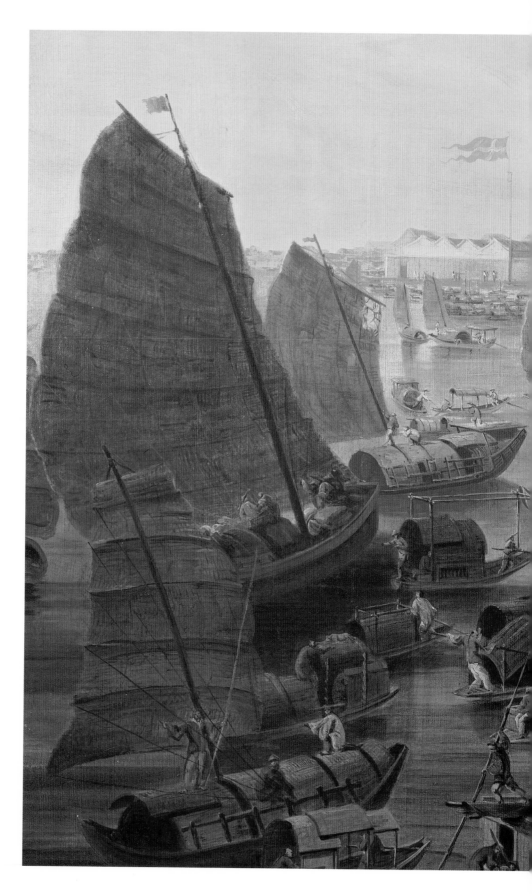

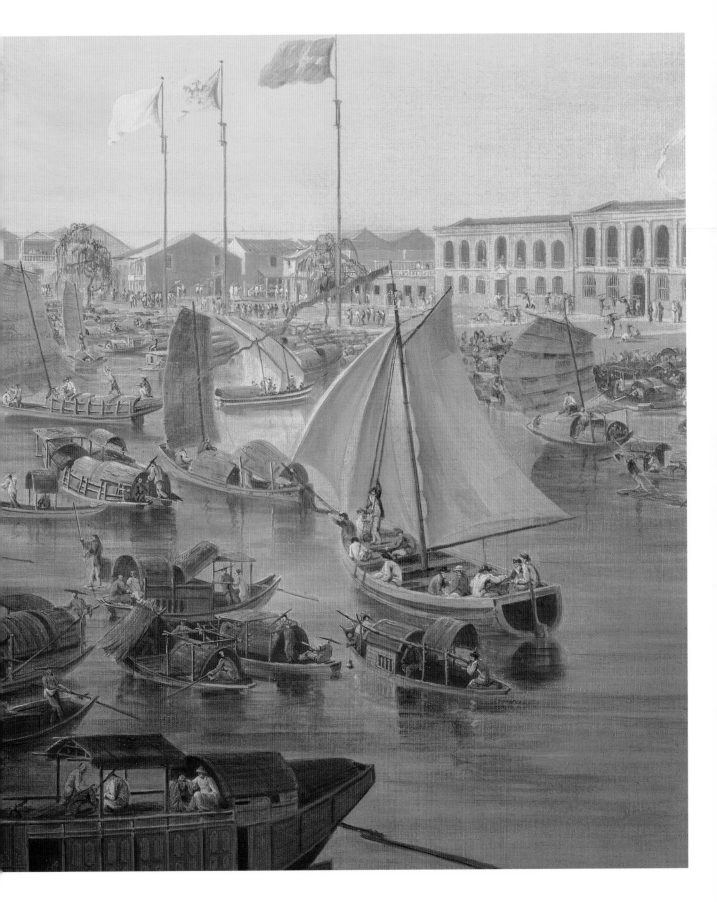

By 1715, China was trying to clean up the opium (called 'Yen' from which the expression 'Having a yen for something' comes) from its shores. In 1729 the Chinese Emperor Yung Ching prohibited the sale of opium and the operating of opium houses. The problem was the conflict in interests between the Chinese government and their merchants who did not really want the goods offered by other trading nations in exchange for the Chinese commodities of rhubarb (used as a laxative by the West), silk and tea. The Chinese preferred Indian opium rather than their own homegrown variety and so the British were able to establish themselves as exporters of opium from India to China by 1780. The drug trade between Britain, India and China then started to bring in huge profits for all those involved. In India alone, the income produced from annual sales of

The Kingdom of China c.1620. The Honourable East India Company had been operating for scarcely a decade when this map was produced.

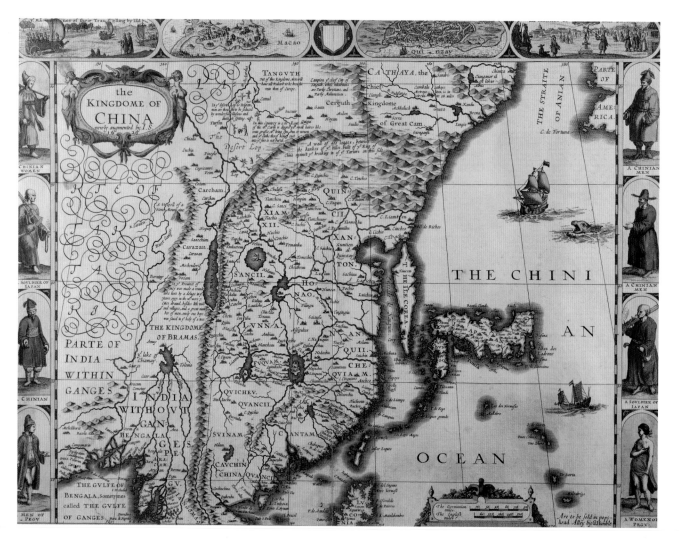

opium, not including inflation, were staggering. In 1840 opium brought in £750,000 but 39 years later opium brought in £9.1 million. The total revenue in this period was £370 million. By comparison today's trade in opium is tiny with total production then of 250,000 tonnes (246,063 tons) compared to the 1999 production of 4,800 tonnes (4,724 tons).

By the nineteenth century, the only trading post open to international trade, or what were deemed 'barbarian' ships, in China was Canton, the capital of Kwangtung province, even though it was technically illegal to offload opium there.

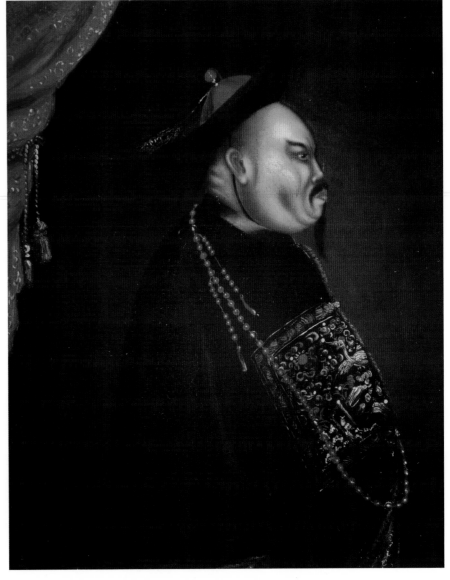

Commissioner Lin, appointed by the Emperor to stamp out the drug trade in Canton.

This was flagrantly ignored with bribes accepted and exchanged on both sides and so the drug trade flourished very quickly. Canton had a reputation for both glamour and squalor with a mix of people endlessly passing through there from all levels of society and cultures. However, the Chinese government were not happy about the spiralling opium trade. There were even threats of cutting out a portion of the upper lips of smokers and other punishments to discourage the trade but laws for foreigners were rarely enforced. In 1839 Commissioner Lin Tse-hau was appointed by the Emperor to clean up Canton. He immediately demanded that the merchants and traders give up their supplies of opium.

This oil on silk painting c.1810 is a revealing early view of Canton. The main square is where the money was negotiated from the sale of opium. Foreign trading houses and the British Hong can be seen in the background.

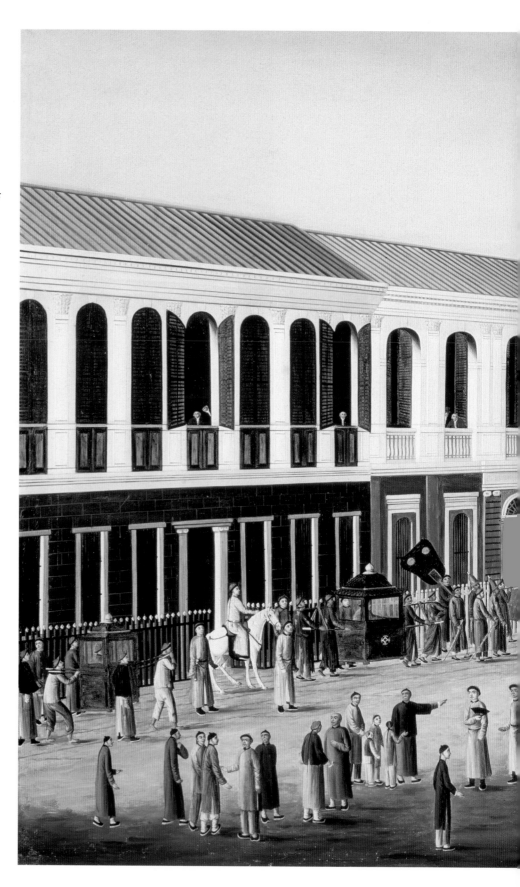

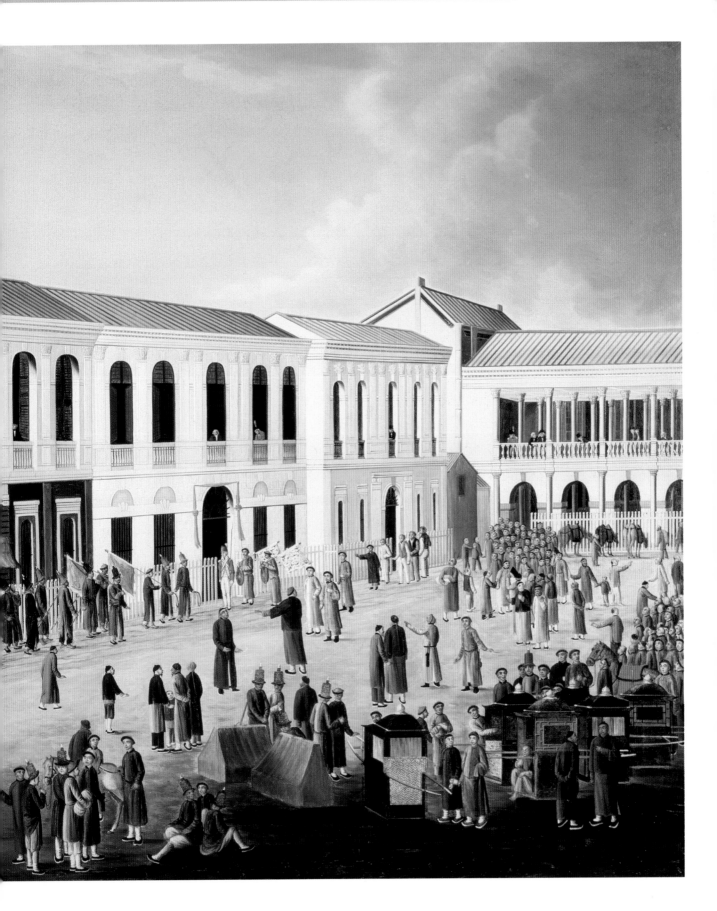

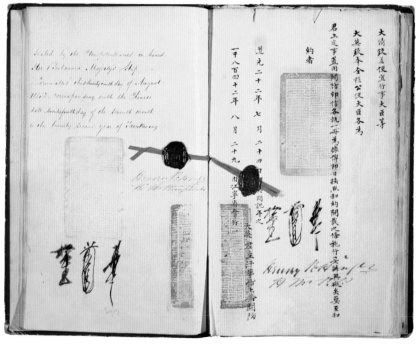

The Treaty of Nanking, agreed between Britain and China after the First Opium War.

Obviously this was met with utter indignation, but Lin was methodical in his workings: opium valued at £6 million was surrendered and destroyed, along with opium pipes and the local crop and so Canton was closed down. This constant aggressive interplay led to the first Opium War between China and Great Britain in 1839 which did not end until 1842. The Chinese could not match the technological and tactical superiority of the British forces. British and European traders refused to stop supplying opium to China until eventually a treaty was signed at Nanking forcing the Chinese to re-open Canton, as well as other ports, to British traders; Hong Kong was ceded to Britain and the Chinese government paid compensation of around £15 million. The French and Americans approached the Chinese after the Nanking Treaty's provisions became known, and in 1844 gained the same trading rights as the British.

It would be a mistake to view the conflict between the two countries simply as a matter of drug control; it was instead the acting-out of deep cultural conflicts between East and West. China's right to rule in its own territory was limited. This began the period referred to by the Chinese as 'the time of unequal treaties'. The British and French again defeated China in a second opium war in 1856. By the terms of the Treaty of Tientsin (1858) the Chinese opened new ports to trading and allowed foreigners with passports to travel in the interior. Christians gained the right to spread their faith and hold property, thus opening up another means of Western penetration. The United States and Russia gained the same privileges in separate treaties. Meanwhile, the opium trade continued to thrive with 15 million reported addicts. Large trading companies like Jardine and Matheson needed to deliver their opium cargoes as quickly as possible to avoid piracy and storms along the China coast and so a new ship was designed: the sleek, fast opium clipper. Usually the clippers offloaded the opium at isolated harbours in exchange for silver.

China, of all the Asian countries, was hardest hit by the evils of opium smoking with the focus of drug traffic moving from Canton to Shanghai. The city became a magnet for cosmopolitan travellers, down-at-heel refugees and petty criminals keen to make a quick fortune but Thailand, Burma, Singapore, Malaysia, Borneo and Vietnam also found themselves caught up in the conflict between condemning the vice and the need for tax revenue from opium. The West discovered, as well, that opium smoking could not be contained in distant colonies; it spread to Europe and North America, adding yet another facet to the world's growing drug problems. Colonialism provided an opportunity for large numbers of Europeans to live beyond their own borders and to adopt exotic manners and customs. With the French settling in North Africa, Southeast Asia and the Middle East, the English in India, Egypt, East Africa and Asia, with the Germans, Belgians, Dutch, Portuguese, Italians and Spanish in their respective colonies, Europe was awash with new ideas. Artisans were

A portrait of Howqua, a distinguished mandarin who encouraged the relationship between East and West, including the trade of opium.

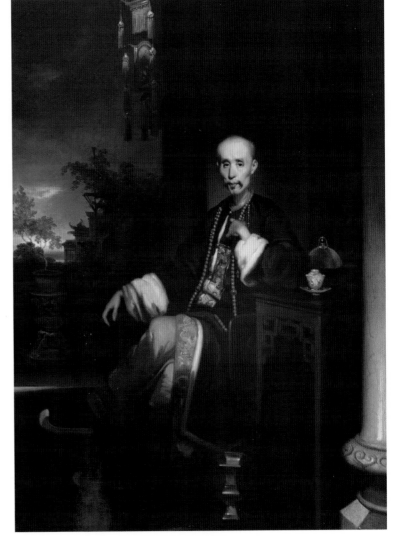

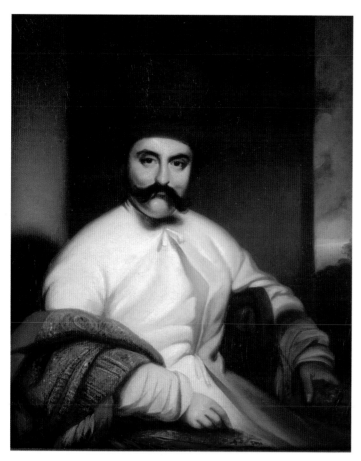

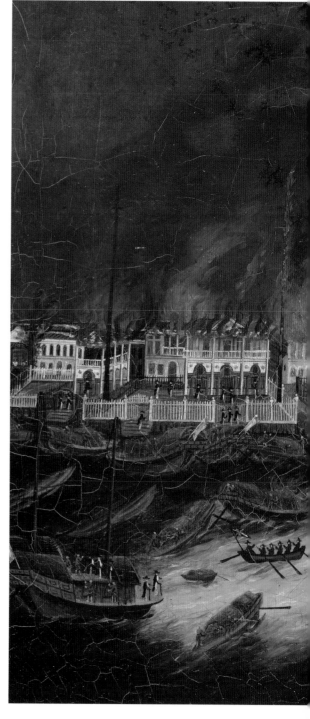

Parsee merchant Sir Jamsetjee Jeejeebhoy, a Knight of the Indian Empire who founded a school of indigenous art in Bombay. Its most famous instructor was Lockwood Kipling, father of Rudyard Kipling.

hired to redecorate the salons of fashionable society in the latest Eastern styles – Chinese, Japanese, Moorish, Indian, Persian, Egyptian. The most famous of these salons to be decorated in these eastern styles was the Prince of Wales's Royal Pavilion in Brighton. Travellers brought back tales of unparalleled danger and rampant sensuality, along with reports of the wealth and grandeur which were at odds with puritanical European ways, yet were attractive because of their exotic strangeness. For those caught in the bleakness of the Industrial Revolution, decadence had never been so appealing. What is now seen by some as a rather suspect

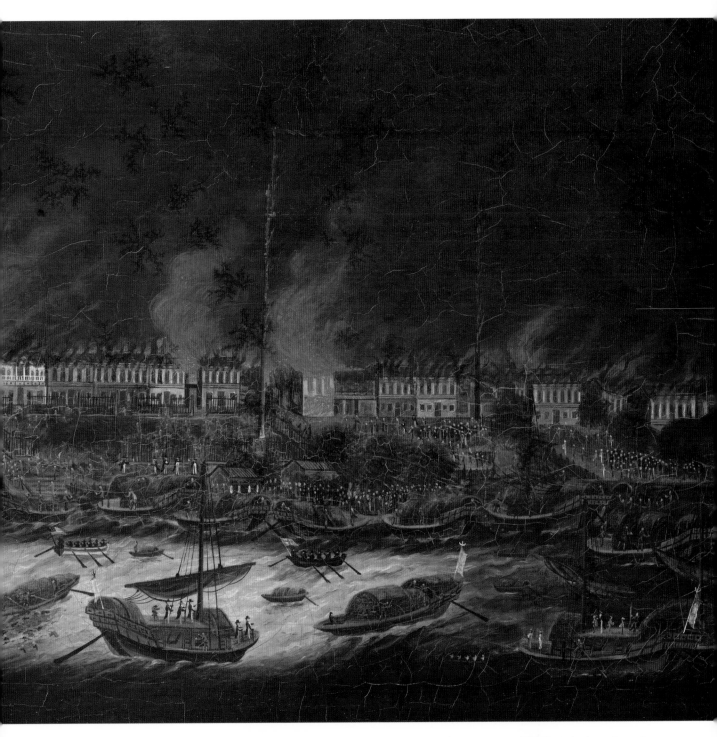

Orientalism was then a breath of fresh air, so when opium smoking was introduced to nineteenth-century Europe by travellers returning from Asia and the Middle East the habit flourished because of a growing passion for the intriguing and exotic ways of the inhabitants of these foreign lands.

The burning of Canton 1822.

OPIUM IN THE WEST IN THE NINETEENTH CENTURY

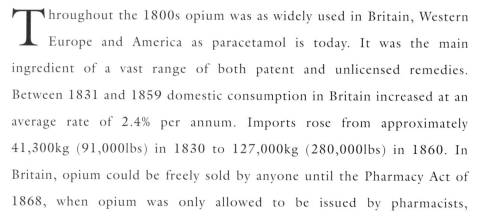

Mowqua acted as middleman between the Western sellers of opium and their Eastern buyers.

hroughout the 1800s opium was as widely used in Britain, Western Europe and America as paracetamol is today. It was the main ingredient of a vast range of both patent and unlicensed remedies. Between 1831 and 1859 domestic consumption in Britain increased at an average rate of 2.4% per annum. Imports rose from approximately 41,300kg (91,000lbs) in 1830 to 127,000kg (280,000lbs) in 1860. In Britain, opium could be freely sold by anyone until the Pharmacy Act of 1868, when opium was only allowed to be issued by pharmacists, although even this did not reduce its availability.

Despite opium production in India, which was largely under British control, most of the importation came from Turkey which manufactured a more potent product. Indian opium had a low morphine content at 5%, whereas Turkish opium had at least 10% morphine content. In Britain, the major ports of Liverpool, Dover and Bristol all traded in opium. London became the main trading centre with the British Levant Company controlling at least 50% of the market destined for Europe and the Americas in the early part of the 1800s. When they closed in 1825 other companies soon took

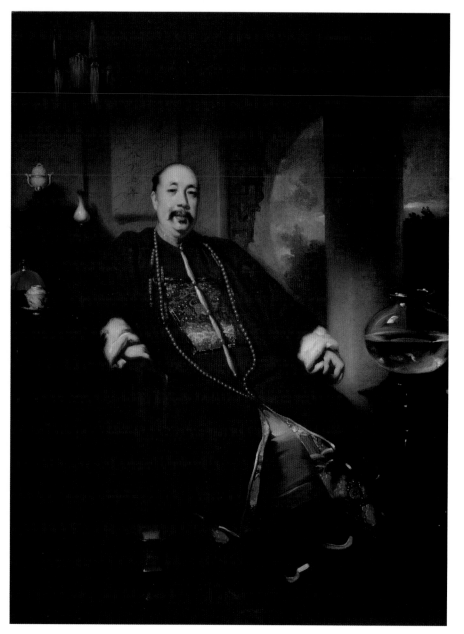

over the wholesale distribution via public and private auction. The centre of the opium business in London was around Mincing Lane, also home to the Tea Exchange. Auctions took place fortnightly and were attended by about 100 buyers and brokers with profits invariably above 50%. Price fluctuations did occur but the British put pressure on foreign governments to encourage their agricultural communities to produce even more, often at the expense of other crops. This meant that the wholesale price did not rise by more than 25% until the twentieth century.

Low-lying areas of France, Holland and Belgium as well as the fenlands which were found on the east coast of England in counties such as Norfolk and Essex, were particularly high in their consumption of opium. This is largely because at that time, there was a large mosquito population, all of whom were vectors in passing diseases such as malaria, which at the time was known as the 'ague'. The mosquitoes thrived in the stagnant pools of the salt marshes and brought discomfort and disease to the surrounding human population. Between 1740 and 1830 attempts were made to grow poppies and harvest opium in Britain, particularly in the fens of Lincolnshire, Norfolk and Cambridgeshire to be used by the local population with chemists eager to cut costs related to import duties. The mild climate found in the south of England yielded better crops although it was mainly a side venture and never went into full-scale production due to the area of land and labour required making it unprofitable. Remedies for malaria often saw opium given in combination with beer and ale or more successfully, in terms of

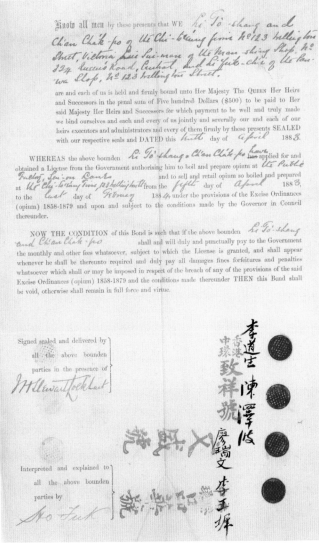

A licence c.1883, granted by the British authorities to legally prepare opium for a period of one year.

reducing mortality rates, with quinine which was extracted from the bark of the South American cinchona tree. In terms of home-grown herbal preparations for children, it was usually the capsule heads of the poppy that were used as they were weaker.

The vast quantities of opium consumed in Britain were not used only by agricultural communities – almost every British person took opium at some time in their lives, including the then Royal Family, and many took it frequently. Mrs Beeton's book *Household Management* written for the upper classes gives a list of remedies, many of which contain opium. However, she was careful to mention her disapproval of its overuse in children when 'Selfish and thoughtless nurses and mothers too, sometimes give cordials and sleeping draughts'. The drug acquired the finest of testimonials. In short, it worked; it was not a placebo as were many medicines and it did away with the need for cupping, bleeding and the application of leeches, all methods which had been used by doctors for centuries. In comparison with these crude treatments opium was gentle. It produced no inconvenience to the patient, save perhaps mild constipation. Indeed it was the first genuine over-the-counter, commercially-produced medicine.

During the first half of the nineteenth century experiments conducted across Europe proved that opium as potent as that of Eastern countries could be produced. In 1830 John Young, a surgeon at Edinburgh, succeeded in obtaining 25kg (56lb) of opium from an acre of poppies. In France the cultivation had been carried on since 1844 at Clermont-Ferrand by Aubergier. The juice evaporated by artificial heat immediately after collection and yielded about one-fourth of its weight of opium, and the percentage of morphine varied according to the variety of poppy used, the purple types giving the best results. Usually anything over 12% was seen as excellent quality. Some specimens of French opium was reported by the pharmacist Guibourt to yield between 12–22.8% of morphine.

Experiments reported by Dietrich in Germany saw opium yields containing from 8%, 13% and again a staggering 22% of morphine. It was found that the method yielding the best results was to make incisions in the poppy-heads soon after sunrise, collect the juice with the finger immediately after incision and evaporate it as speedily as possible, the colour of the opium being lighter and the percentage of morphine greater than when the juice was allowed to dry on the plant. Cutting through the poppy-head caused the shrivelling-up of the young fruit, but the heads which had been carefully incised yielded more seed than those which had not been cut at all. The giant variety of poppy yielded the most morphine. The experiments were never developed to full-scale production as it was far cheaper to import opium due to the land and labour required.

In 1806 a 21-year-old German pharmacist's assistant, Friedrich Sertürner, was to alter the future of medicine. His careful experimentation resulted in the discovery of morphine. He prophetically wrote 'I consider it my duty to attract attention to the terrible effects of this new substance in order that calamity may be averted.' At first, because of his lack of formal qualifications, his work was ignored but a French chemist, Gay-Lussac, drew attention to it. In 1821 the Institute of France awarded Sertürner a prize and citation for having 'opened the way to important medical discoveries by his isolation of morphine and his exposition of its character', and so in the early 1820s morphine was made available on a commercial basis throughout Western Europe, closely followed by America.

In 1874 at St Mary's Hospital, Paddington, London a pharmacist called C.R. Alder Wright conducted experiments in order to find a non-addictive alternative to morphine and in 1887 several papers were published following up on his work identifying the newly named diacetylmorphine as a narcotic more potent than morphine. Its singular molecular structure was proven in 1890 but it was not until 1898 when the German chemist, Heinrich Dresser, working for the Bayer laboratories produced a quantity of

Hong Kong in the 1840s showing the extensive and impressive growth of the city following the Treaty of Nanking.

diacetylmorphine. After clinical trials it proved to be a hugely powerful painkiller. Bayer then mass-marketed it under a brand name based upon the German word 'heroish' meaning heroic and it was subsequently named Heroin.

It might have seemed like everyone was taking opiates but the great social problems opium caused, both here and abroad, did not go unnoticed. The link between mosquitoes and malaria was finally understood. Eradication programmes in the fenlands started to reduce mosquito numbers and disease rates declined accordingly. Temperance societies sprang up and in 1874 the Society for the Suppression of the Opium Trade was formed by a group of concerned Quakers. Other groups interested in social reform soon joined and the tide began to turn.

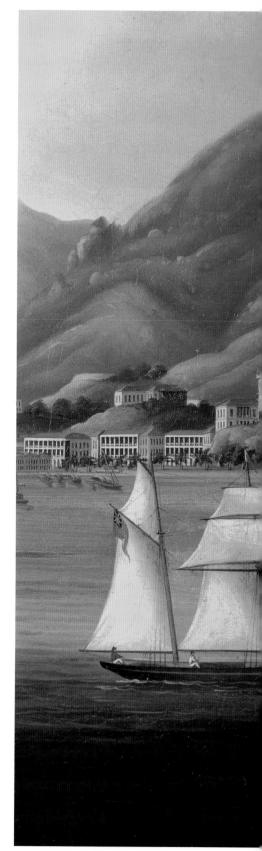

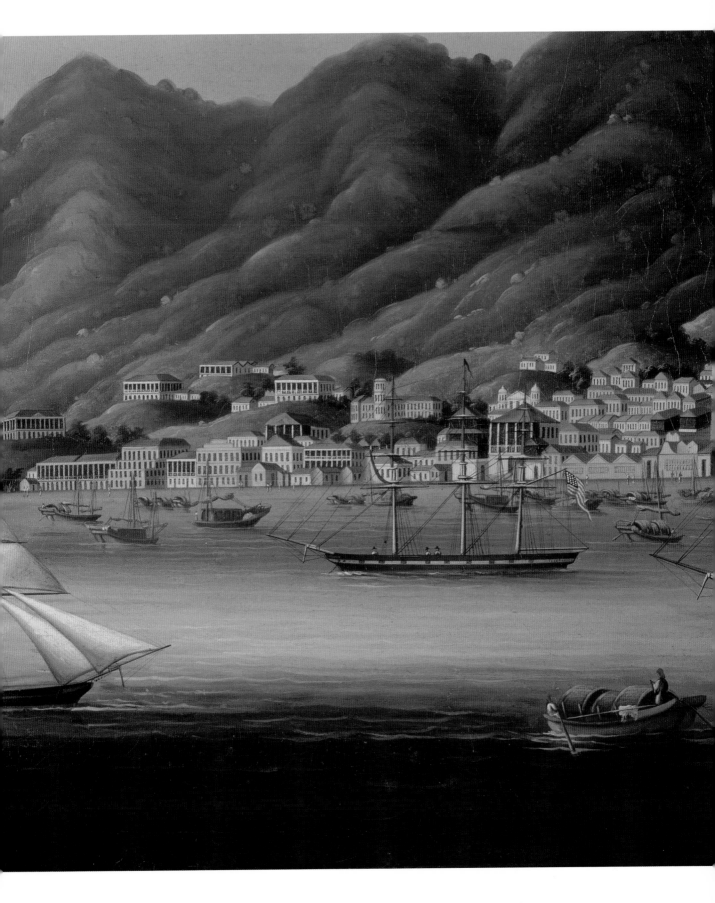

OPIUM IN THE TWENTIETH CENTURY

The US-based Saint James Society mounted a campaign to supply free samples of heroin through mail order to morphine addicts who were trying to come off opium. The results were of course unsuccessful. However, around the same time, the British and French were trying to control opium production in Southeast Asia. This worked to an extent, but the Southeast region, the 'Golden Triangle', was still producing large quantities of the drug and during the 1940s became one of the major suppliers of opium. Various medical journals reported side effects of using heroin as a cure for morphine addiction. Many physicians argued that their patients would suffer from heroin withdrawal symptoms equal to that of morphine addiction: regardless of the warnings, heroin addiction rose steadily.

New York's Chinatown became infamous for drug dealers in the 1930s. Illegal heroin was smuggled into the US from China and was refined in Shanghai and Tientsin. During the Second World War, the opium trade routes became blocked and the flow of opium from India and Persia was cut off. In 1945–7 Burma gained her independence from Britain at the end of the war and unfortunately opium cultivation and trade flourished in the Shan states. The availability of opium increased by a huge percentage. Dealers and addicts alike were easily able to get their hands on the drug that was being smuggled into the US. It was at this time that the Burmese officially outlawed opium.

By the 1950s and into the 1970s, Mafia-controlled drug distributors began to dominate the US heroin market through Corsican gangsters (the 'French Connection'). After refining the raw Turkish opium in Marseille laboratories, the heroin was made easily available for purchase by addicts on New York City streets. The US efforts to contain the spread of Communism in Asia involved making alliances with various tribes and warlords inhabiting the areas of the Golden Triangle, thus began a complicated set of allegiances. In order to maintain their relationship with the warlords while continuing to fund the struggle against communism, the US and France supplied the drug warlords and their armies with ammunition, arms and air transport for the production and sale of opium.

Smuggled opium sealed in waxy paper.

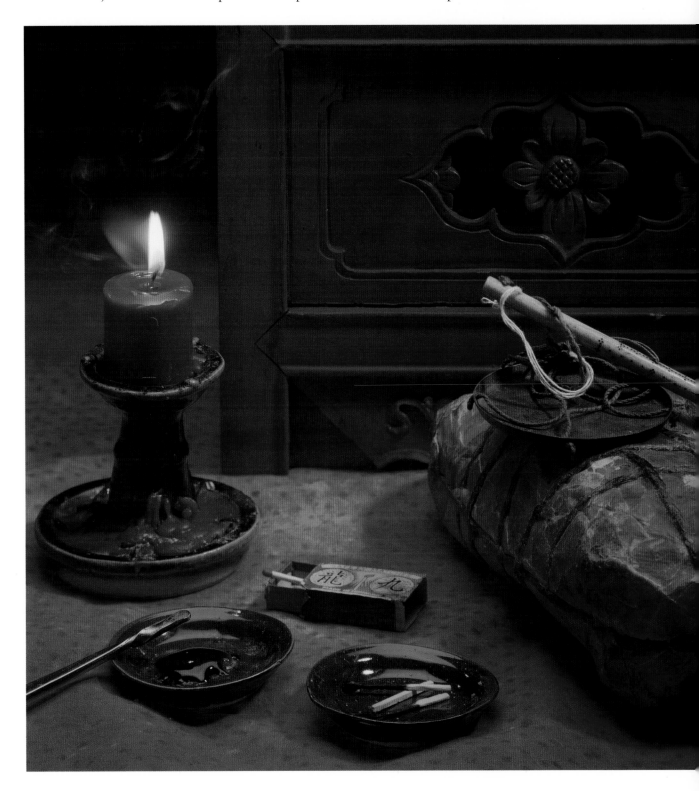

45

Right: Raw opium in its moisturising banana leaf being weighed on a traditional Chinese scale.

One of the after-effects of the Vietnam War was the surge in illegal heroin smuggling into the US. The US was blamed for allowing it to happen, and for utilising the Central Intelligence Agency (CIA) to set up a charter airline, Air America, to transport raw opium from Burma and Laos. At this time, the number of heroin addicts in the US reached an estimated 750,000. The Shan warlord, Khun Sa, was controlling the South-east Asia's Golden Triangle and was making a huge amount of money in the opium trade. The other source of heroin coming into the USA was Mexico. Eventually in 1973 President Nixon created the DEA (Drug Enforcement Administration) under the Justice Department to consolidate virtually all federal powers of drug enforcement into a single agency. By the time Saigon fell in the mid-1970s, the US and Mexican governments were working on a way to destroy the main source of raw opium. This was done by spraying poppy fields with a chemical called Agent Orange. It halted the flow of one type of heroin, 'Mexican Mud' but this was soon replaced by another generation of heroin, this time from Afghanistan which until recently produced 90% of the world's opium with Pakistan 5%, and Turkey and Colombia 2% each.

'I took a line that comes from the golden states of Shan
The smugglers trail that leads to the opium den
The Chinese connection refines to heroin
Depart the heart you crave again'

Opium Trail by Thin Lizzy (1971)

It was only the hospice movement of the mid twentieth century for terminally-ill cancer patients that now saw opium and the opiates derived from it as being a blessing.

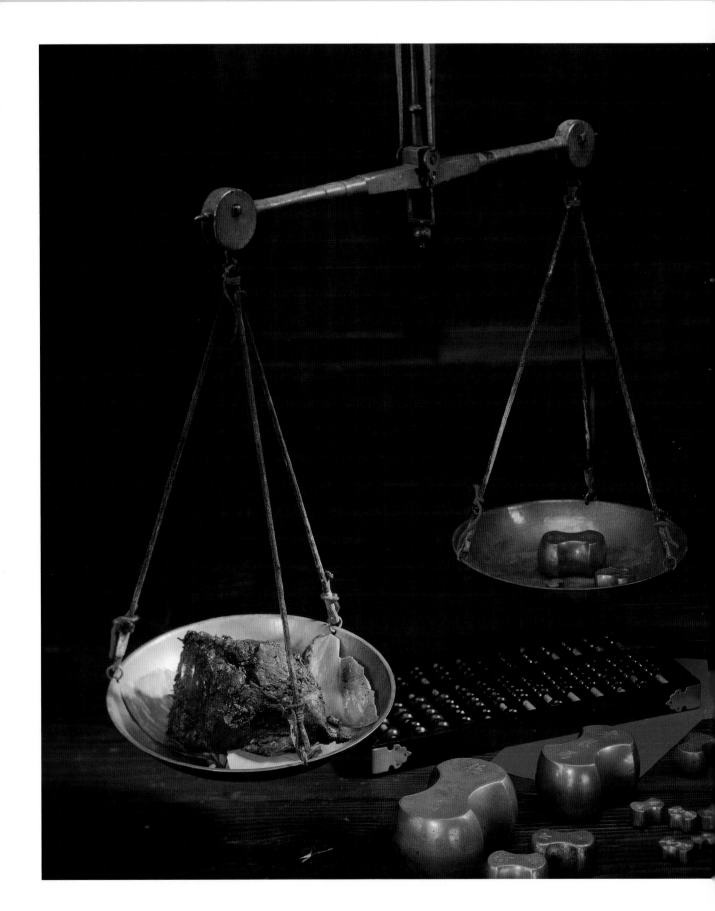

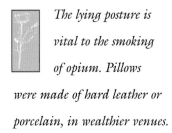

The lying posture is vital to the smoking of opium. Pillows were made of hard leather or porcelain, in wealthier venues.

Prior to the Second World War, all countries in South-east Asia had state-controlled opium monopolies, similar in many ways to the tobacco monopolies which are prevalent today. Most local addicts were ethnic Chinese who had migrated into South-east Asia's urban centres, bringing with them their opium-smoking habits. Despite this ready market, there was hardly any poppy cultivation in this area until the 1940s; prior to this perhaps 30 tonnes (29.5 tons) a year were grown in the Shan Hills. When the Second World War broke out many of the trade routes from India and Persia were blocked. The French began to expand into new territories to ensure their opium trade was not lost. The Shan area, north of Thailand and between Burma, Yunnan and French Indo-China was too politically and ethnically diverse to become a separate-run territory of British India. The area was run by dozens of different princes and they were encouraged by the French to ensure local farmers grew opium which in turn saw the princes achieved comfortable incomes from taxes imposed.

In 1950, after the Chinese revolution, hundreds of defeated Nationalist troops from Yunnan province in China fled across the border into the Shan territory, to escape their Communist oppressors. By 1953 there were over 12,000 based there. The Burmese Army failed to defeat them in battle but many of the survivors moved into the opium-growing area of the Shan states and the era of the warlords began. In order to finance its secret war against the Communists in China, the nationalist troops persuaded the hill tribe farmers to grow more opium and then introduced a heavy opium tax which forced them to grow even more in order to make ends meet. By the mid-1950s, opium production in the Golden Triangle had reached 500 tonnes (492 tons) per annum and a large percentage was being exported to the USA. The CIA, eager to protect their own country, began clandestine operations against the warlords but failed. In 1959, the Shan princes renounced all their powers and handed over to a democratically-elected Shan Government. The territory was now known as Shan State.

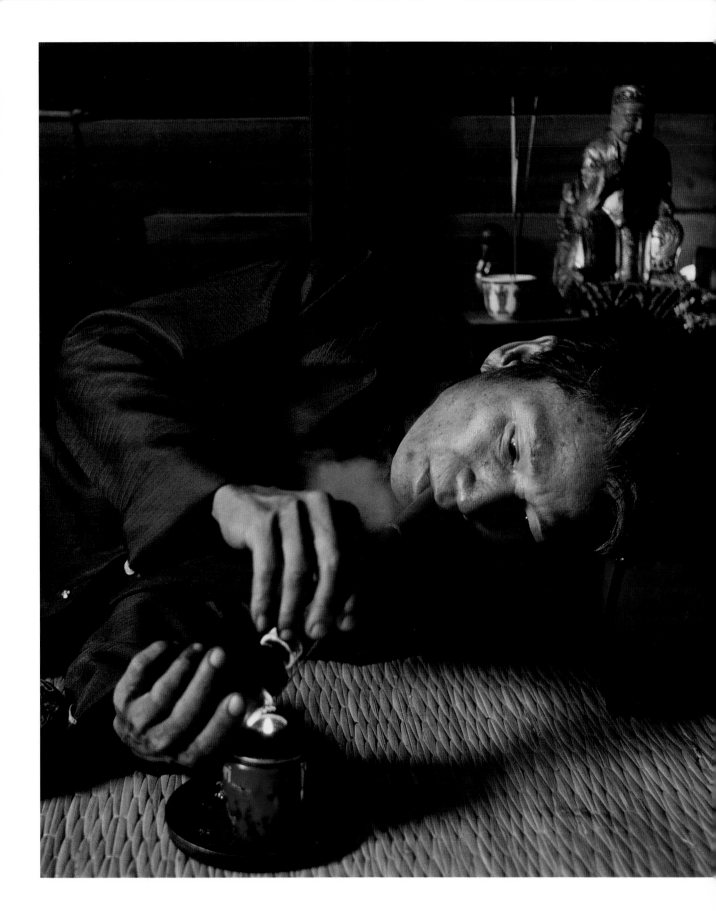

In order to finance their defence, the opium warlords now moved into a new area of profitability by importing skilled chemists from Hong Kong and Taiwan to turn their raw opium into morphine and later heroin, as this was where the profits were really being made. South-east Asia's first heroin refineries were established in the mid-1960s. In 1962, there was a coup and Shan State was thrown into anarchy. The revitalised People's Army of Burma forced the Nationalist warlords to retreat to the Thai border. At the border, these 'regiments' established tax stations where they collected customs duty on opium convoys entering Thailand.

By the late 1960s the emerging opium hierarchy consisted first of the farmers who grew the poppies and who earned a pittance for months of laborious work. Despite living at subsistence level they had to pay taxes to various rebel groups in their area. These rebels also received taxes from the merchants who bought the opium from the farmers. The merchants were respectable businessmen who were licensed to sell opium quite openly at local markets. The merchants hired mercenaries to guard their convoys which took the opium to the market town of Tachilek, near the border junction between Burma, Laos and Thailand. There the opium was exchanged for bars of pure gold, hence the area's nickname 'The Golden Triangle'. The mercenary commanders then purchased consumer goods using the gold which they took back as a return cargo, which they in turn sold to the merchants who in turn sold back to the farmers. Some of this return cargo was used as bribes for government and civilian officials as well as military officers in order for them to turn a blind eye to the opium harvest. Alongside this the CIA used as many contacts as they could gain as their own intelligence assets and recruited mercenaries with the armies of the warlords to fight another secret war against North Vietnamese troops and local communists in Laos. The opium then moved from Tachilek to the heroin refineries along the Thai–Burma border which were owned by ethnic Chinese connected to the Triads, who in turn moved the heroin through a series of couriers all

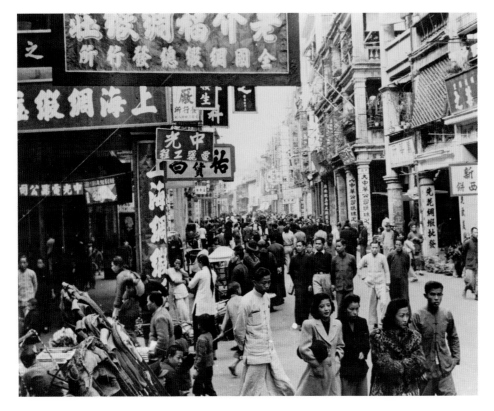

Although most of the narcotics from the Golden Triangle were destined for foreign markets, drug abuse is still widespread in the Golden Triangle, with an addiction rate as high as 80% of all males.

over the world. The final link in the chain were the addicts and their families who, next to the impoverished farmers, were without doubt the most pitiable victims of the opium trade. Although most of the narcotics from the Golden Triangle were destined for foreign markets, drug abuse is still widespread in the villages of the Golden Triangle itself, with an addiction rate as high as 80% of all males. After President Nixon launched his war on drugs in the 1970s, millions of dollars were funnelled into the hill tribe economy of the Golden Triangle in order to provide the opium farmers with substitute crops.

During the early 1970s most of the heroin that was entering the USA was coming from Asia and Turkey via France, particularly through the French port of Marseilles, where it was also being refined. The smuggling operation was run by French-Corsican mafia, and was famously christened 'The French Connection'. Fortunately, because the operation was so centralised, once it was known about by the American law enforcement agencies, a plan of attack was launched and it was for the most part shut down.

Gold opium in china ramekins, exotic and alluring. Opium is often stored in the crush-proof packaging originally designed and produced for cigarettes; easy to carry away and hide in the event of a police raid.

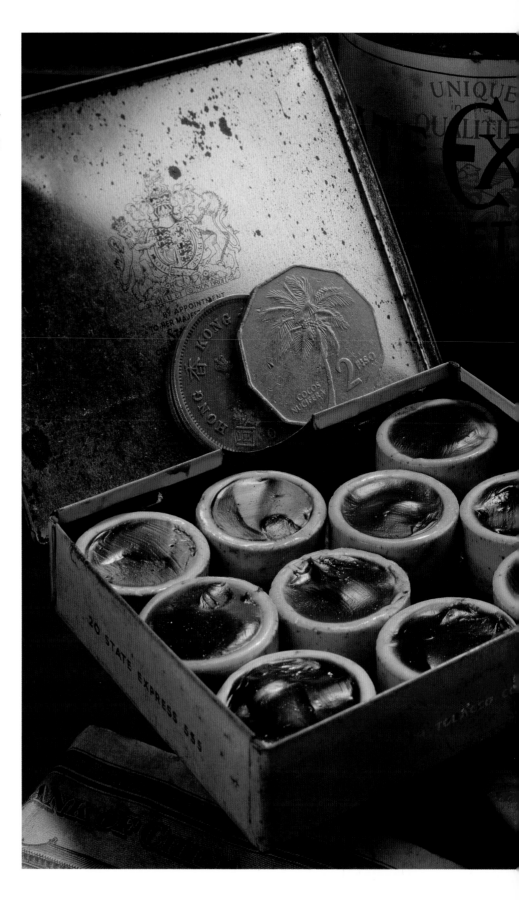

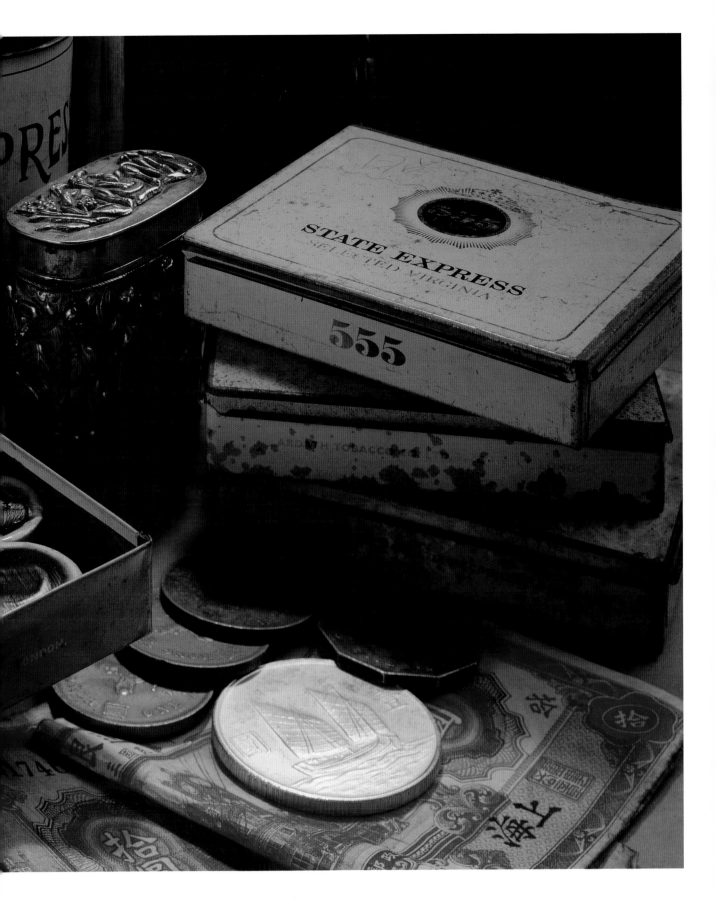

In recent years, the UK has accounted for the greatest proportion of heroin seized in Western Europe. At the beginning of the Millennium over 3,000kg (6,615lbs) of heroin was seized, which was 44% up on seizures from 1999. In 1999 illegal opium production rose significantly due to the record harvest in Afghanistan. Global production of opium that year was 4,800 tonnes (4,724 tons), which was sufficient to produce around 480 tonnes (472 tons) of heroin, of which the UK consumed 10%. Due to the fundamentalist Taliban regime in Afghanistan, who were in the process of destroying the opium fields, opium exports fell dramatically towards the end of their regime to around 180 tonnes (177 tons), when they outlawed its production on religious grounds. Of the heroin seized in the UK, 90% has its origins in Afghanistan. The remaining 10% can be traced back to Burma and Laos.

The people of Afghanistan have suffered tremendously under various regime changes through the late twentieth century. In the 1970s the country was overrun with communism and freedom fighters called the mujhadeen tried to oust them. The latter groups were originally funded through drug money, particularly opium sales, and encouraged by the American CIA whose policy was to encourage them to ensure that they had the weapons to attack the Russian troops.

Conversion to morphine and heroin mainly takes places in the neighbouring countries of South-west Asia, but increasingly in Afghanistan itself. It has been suggested by some analysts that there may be a gap of some two years between the planting of an opium crop and the purchase of heroin in the UK. Part of the period is taken up with the planting, growing and then harvesting of opium, its conversion to morphine and then to heroin. The heroin is then stored, awaiting transportation to its destination and is often stockpiled en route.

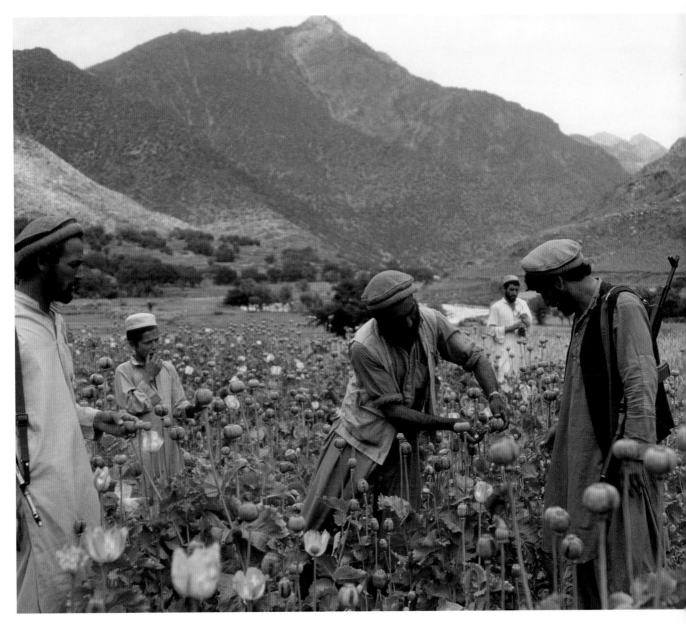

The drugs are then transported via Iran, Pakistan, Turkey and the Central Asian republics and then along the Balkan route, where Anglo-Turkish organised crime groups control its sale and distribution. Heroin enters the UK in freight and vehicles, predominantly in ports in southern and eastern England but recent Home Office reports are showing that new routes are opening up through the Caucasus into Russia and then Poland, a route further exacerbated by the fall of the Eastern Bloc and the take-over by the Russian mafia. The annual number of seizures involving heroin rose continually over the last decade.

Opium harvest in Afghanistan.

55

The United Nation Office for Drug Control and Crime Prevention has conducted an annual opium poppy survey in Afghanistan since 1994. The results provide a detailed picture of each year's season. During the 1990s Afghanistan firmly established itself as the largest source of illicit opium and heroin in the world. By the end of the 1990s Afghanistan provided about 70% of global illicit opium production. Myanmar (Burma) produced about 22% and Laos about 3%. Illicit opiates of Afghan origin were consumed by an estimated 9 million, which is two-thirds of all opiate users in the world. It is estimated that along the trafficking chain about half-a-million people have been involved in the trade of illicit Afghan opiates in recent years. The overall turnover of this illicit trade from Afghanistan is estimated to be US$25 billion per annum. The power vacuum in Kabul caused by the aftermath of 9/11 and the subsequent war in Afghanistan enabled farmers to replant the opium poppy plants that had been destroyed by the Taliban regime. Because of the conflict on the ground following 9/11, the field work of United Nations Drug Control and Crime Prevention department ceased and the recent survey had to be based on high-resolution satellite images, owing to the instability of the region, which were able to identify poppy fields in about 600 locations with a total area estimated around 70,000 hectares. The average opium yield is estimated at 46kg (101lbs) per hectare giving a total of 3,400 tonnes (3,346 tons).

'From wandering through a many-solemn scene
Of opium visions, with a heart serene
And intellect miraculously bright;
I wake from daydreams to this real night'

The City of Dreadful Night
by James Thomson (1834–82)

'The prestige of government has undoubtedly been lowered considerably by the Prohibition law. For nothing is more destructive of respect for the government and the law of the land than passing laws which cannot be enforced. It is an open secret that the dangerous increase of crime in this country is closely connected with this.'

Albert Einstein (1879–1955)

Opium has only been illegal for a short period of its history. From being a 'Gift of the Gods' and a vital component of medicine, its use for purely social purposes made it intolerable as it brought down whole sections of society. In Britain the Pharmacy Act was introduced in 1868 which made opium only available through the medical profession due to the machinations of the Pharmaceutical Society. In 1905 the United States Congress banned opium. The next year, China and England finally designed a treaty restricting the Sino-Indian opium trade. Physicians at this time experimented with treatments for heroin addiction. In 1906 the US Congress passed the Pure Food and Drug Act requiring contents labelling on patent medicines by pharmaceutical companies. Opium use as an ingredient in these medicines started to decline by 1909 as public awareness was raised. The United States was also pressing for legislation aimed at suppressing the sale of opium to China. On February 1st 1909, The International Opium Commission met in Shanghai with Dr. Hamilton Wright and Episcopal Bishop Henry Brent heading the US delegation. Their job was to try to convince the international delegation of the negative and destructive effects of opium. By 1910, and after nearly 150 years of failed attempts to rid the country of opium, the Chinese were finally successful in convincing the British to end the India–China opium trade.

Opium stored in snuffboxes, cigar humidors and tobacco pouches.

In 1914 the Harrison Narcotics Act was passed; this aimed to curb abuse and addiction. It required doctors, pharmacists and others who prescribed narcotics to register and pay a tax. The US government made a number of attempts to halt the growing drug problem. A committee on drug addiction was formed in 1921 and the Narcotic Drugs Import and Export Act of 1922 increased penalties and established a Federal Narcotics Control Board. Congress effectively outlawed all domestic use and production of heroin in 1924 and in 1927 the Bureau of Prohibition was formed. By 1923 the US Treasury Department's Narcotics Division banned all legal narcotics sales. This forced addicts to buy from black-market suppliers. In 1929 the Rockefeller Foundation in tandem with government agencies began a research programme to find non-addictive substitutes for morphine-based drugs. It was hoped that a synthetic version of morphine could be created without negative side effects.

In 1968 the Bureau of Narcotics and Dangerous Drugs was established in the US with international responsibilities and contacts. In 1970 the Drug Abuse Prevention and Control Act came into force along with the Controlled Substances Act. During the 1970s the DEA had astounding success which resulted in the US addict population dropping from 500,000 to 200,000. However, during the 1980s it rose to such a high level that a new law, the Drug Abuse Act of 1986, gave the police force increased powers against dealers. In 1989 the situation became so bad that President Bush announced a $7.8 billion programme declaring war on Latin American drug cartels.

In 1971 the Misuse of Drugs Act was passed in the UK. This meant that drugs were given classifications. Opium, morphine, methadone, pethidine, diconal and heroin are all treated as Class A drugs, which are the most serious in legal terms. This means that for possession an offender can expect seven years imprisonment, a heavy fine or both. A person who is found guilty of supplying the drug can expect a life sentence, a heavy fine or both.

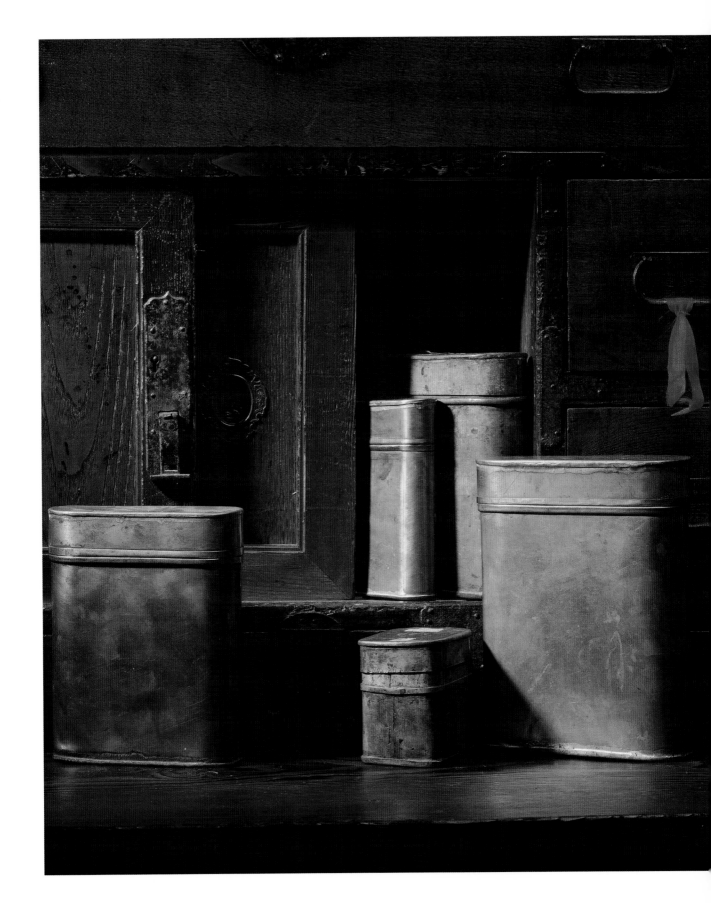

THE UNITED NATIONS AND OPIUM

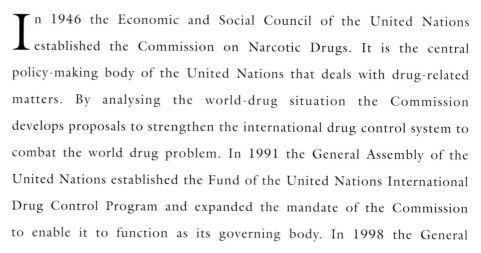

Bernard Frahi, representative of the United Nations Drug Control Program, shows the World Drug Report 2000 to reporters during a news conference.

In 1946 the Economic and Social Council of the United Nations established the Commission on Narcotic Drugs. It is the central policy-making body of the United Nations that deals with drug-related matters. By analysing the world-drug situation the Commission develops proposals to strengthen the international drug control system to combat the world drug problem. In 1991 the General Assembly of the United Nations established the Fund of the United Nations International Drug Control Program and expanded the mandate of the Commission to enable it to function as its governing body. In 1998 the General Assembly passed a mandate devoted to countering the world drug problem and further strengthened its role as the global forum for international co-operation in combating the world drug problem and its functions as the governing body of UNDCP.

Drug abuse is a global phenomenon and affects almost every country, although its extent and characteristics are different from region to region. Drug abuse trends throughout the world, especially among the young, have started to converge over the last few years. Three-quarters of all countries report abuse of heroin. Drug-related problems include increased rate of crime and violence as well as increased susceptibility to infectious diseases such as HIV/AIDS and Hepatitis, demand for treatment in emergency room visits which put strain on health services, and a breakdown in social behaviour.

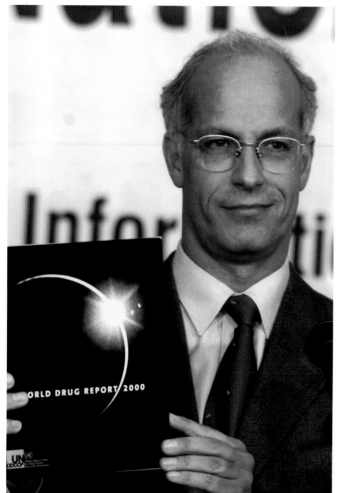

ORLD DRUG REPORT 2000

Demand-reduction strategies set up by the UNODC seek to prevent the onset of drug use, help drug users break the habit and provide treatment through rehabilitation and social integration. At the 1998 UN General Assembly Special Session on the World Drug Problem, member states recognised that reducing the demand for drugs was an essential pillar in the stepped-up global effort to fight drug abuse and trafficking. They committed themselves to reduce significantly both the supply of and demand for drugs by 2008. Reducing the supply and availability of illicit drugs is the other essential component in the fight against drug abuse. UNODC Projects seek to limit the cultivation, production, trafficking and distribution of drugs. Efforts to reduce the supply of drugs included encouraging those farmers who cultivate illicit crops such as opium to switch to other profitable crops and alternative sources of income. This goal is achieved through alternative development projects, community development, natural resource management and income-generating projects. Supply-reduction projects also seek to broaden regional co-operation between governments in response to cross-border trafficking by strengthening border controls and providing them with modern equipment and training in law enforcement procedures. By improving the socio-economic quality of life of targeted populations through integrated development projects, UNODC seeks to prevent, reduce and eliminate the production of illicit drug crops. Comprehensive alternative development projects address the broader economic situation of farmers who cultivate drug crops due to rural poverty and a lack of access to markets for legal products and unsuitable soil for many other crops. UNODC Law Enforcement Section ensures a uniformity of approach and the application of best practices in all projects containing a law enforcement component. It acts as a liaison between its international law enforcement partners such as the World Customs Organisation and Interpol.

Due to the efforts of this organisation, Pakistan was virtually poppy-free in the year 2000, production having been all but eradicated following the implementation of a 15-year United Nations programme. Opium cultivation in Laos has been cut by 30% and in Vietnam it has been cut by 90%. The global area under opium poppy cultivation is at its lowest level since 1998. The profile of illegal drugs in the economies of the main-producing countries has seen a decisive trend of decline. During the 1990s consumption trends of the main problem drugs in the developed countries has been stable or in decline. China, for so long synonymous with the production and consumption of opium itself, succeeded in eradicating opium between 1949 and 1954. At the height of its problem China had over 20 million opium addicts, which is more than the approximately 14 million worldwide addicts today. In the UK alone it is estimated that beyond the 40,000 registered addicts there are another 100,000 unregistered users.

At present the British government is overseeing the United Nations Strategy to eliminate the opium crop in Afghanistan. The plan includes working with a coalition of countries on the borders of Afghanistan in order to introduce an integrated strategy to reduce trafficking. At present the British government's policy is to pay the farmers a subsidy depending on the amount of hectares they have under opium production. Unfortunately this strategy is unsuccessful because the farmers are growing even more poppies in order to gain larger subsidies. There was a wasted opportunity to destroy all opium during the occupation by Allied forces in the same way that the Taliban did.

Also no policy can stop the farmers being threatened by organised crime. The farmer gets the same amount of money regardless of what they are growing; it is only up the chain that the profits start to be accrued. The warlords of the Northern Alliance, who were our allies during the Afghan War, now control the harvest and trafficking again. Because over 60% of the road network in Afghanistan was destroyed during the war, thereby curtailing an easy access to markets for legal produce, the willingness of middlemen to buy opium poppies at the farm gate, thereby eliminating the transport worry, represents even further incentive for farmers to cultivate the opium poppy crop. There is a four-year UN Alternative Development Project in Nangarhar and Quandahar to find replacement crops for opium farmers to grow, as well as a programme of job creation for the itinerant harvesters.

Taliban destroying a crop of opium poppies.

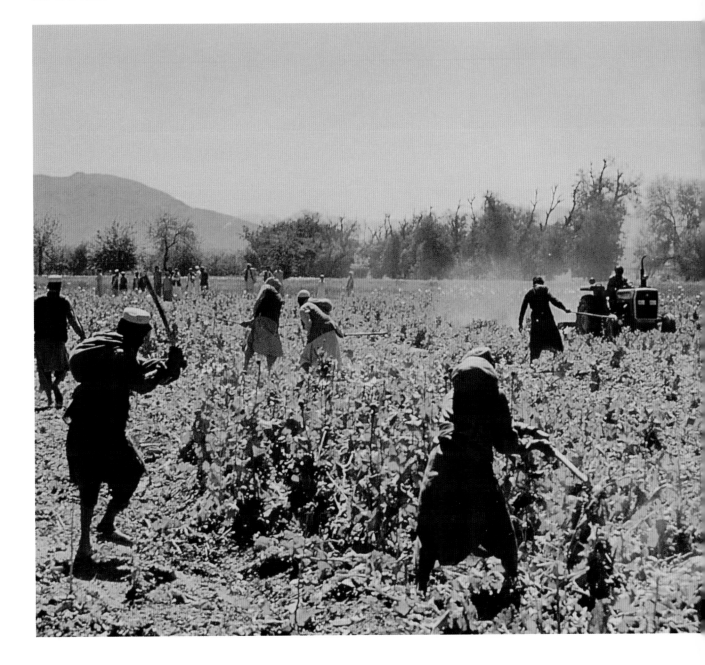

'And now, my beauties! Something with poison in it I think. With poison in it, but attractive to the eye and soothing to the smell ... poppies, poppies, poppies!'

The Wicked Witch of the West in the film
***The Wizard of Oz* (1939)**

To most of us, poppies are the scarlet blooms that we associate with Remembrance Day growing around the makeshift graves of soldiers in the First World War. In fact the opium poppy is part of a family of over 250 species. There are many varieties including the Syrian Tulip Poppy, the Welsh Poppy and the Syrian Blue and all come in a variety of beautiful colours as well as petal forms. All poppies are hypogynous, that is, the reproductive organs of the flower are located under the base of the ovary.

Only the opium poppy, Papaver somniferum Linnaeus, yields enough opium to be used for commercial purposes. It is an annual plant with a growth cycle of around 120 days. In order to grow it requires rich, well-cultivated soil. It seems to grow well in farmland, perhaps because the soil has been recently ploughed and is nutrient-rich, making this kind of soil softer and easier for the plant to root. The best growing climate is fairly warm (minimum 15° C) with low humidity and not too much rainfall during early growth. If there is too much rain, the soil may become waterlogged, especially if it does not have good drainage. If there is not enough rain, the plant will dry out and the opium yield will be seriously affected. Sunlight is especially important. The opium poppy will not bloom unless it has grown through a period of long days and short nights, preferably with direct sunlight at least twelve hours daily. However, as long as climactic conditions are good, the opium plant is fairly easy to grow; it does not have many pest-related problems and needs little tending.

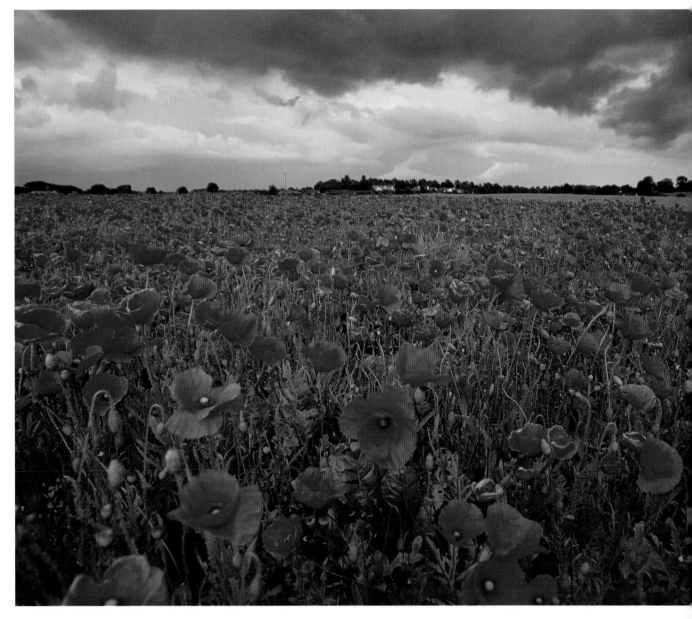

The seeds sow themselves as the poppy head sways in the breeze. One seed pod may produce over 1,000 seeds, although seed heads have been found with as many as 30,000 seeds. They range over a wide variety of colours from white through yellow to brown, grey or black, but the colour of the seed does not affect the colour of the bloom of the poppy. They are often grown alongside other crops. It takes six weeks for the plant to really establish itself. At this point it is not as attractive as it will be in full bloom, looking like a young cabbage with a blue-grey tinge. Occasionally opium poppies can be found growing in gardens of people

A field of red poppies.

65

who are not aware of what they are. Indeed many gardeners presume they are going to be getting a cabbage crop if poppies have self-seeded on their property without them knowing.

At eight weeks it reaches a height of 60cm (23.6in). It has a main stem which is usually covered in fine hairs. The topmost part is called the peduncle and this has no leaves or secondary stems. Secondary stems grow from below the peduncle and these are called tillers. The plant matures to a height of around 90–150cm (35.4–59in). Long rectangular serrated-edged leaves appear alternately. On the main stem each tiller extends into a single flower bud which eventually will bloom into the flower, although before this happens they droop into a hook shape. The colour varies from pink to crimson to white. Inside the bloom is a ring of anthers. These later become the top of the pod, or crown. This beautiful but fragile bloom only lasts for around four days, then the petals drop off, leaving the pod sack exposed. As this grows, it can reach the size of a small chicken egg. When the pod is ready the crown exposes holes, like a pepperpot, that allow the seeds to fall out. The seeds are edible but the trace of opium is so small that you would never be able to detect it in a normal diet. There are no known side-effects to eating them and they are considered legal in most countries. The opium sap itself is quite different. It has several components including proteins, sugars, ammonia, latex, gums, fats, sulphuric and lactic acids, plant wax, water, meconic acid and a wide range of alkaloids. The smell of fresh opium sap is bitter but pungent due to the presence of these alkaloids.

Opium works by replacing the natural painkillers that exist in the human brain. These are called opiate peptides and they include enkephalins, dynophins and endorphins. Unfortunately, after a few weeks of continuous opium use, the body stops producing these natural pain inhibitors which is why withdrawal is so painful for the user. Endorphins are also responsible for making us feel happy, which means that depression and anxiety take hold as soon as the drug is taken away. An alkaloid is a highly complex organic base (an alkali) with the common characteristic properties of containing nitrogen, of being basic and forming salts and water with acids, found in plants and having a characteristically bitter taste. Over 50 have been identified in opium, the most important being morphine (from which heroin can be made) noscapine, papaverine, codeine and thebaine. They appear partially or loosely chemically bonded to meconic acid, the presence of which can be used as a test to detect opium. It is not known why the plant has evolved in this way, some theories suggesting that it has developed its alkaloid bitterness as some sort of deterrent to hungry animals, but it remains an enigma to this day.

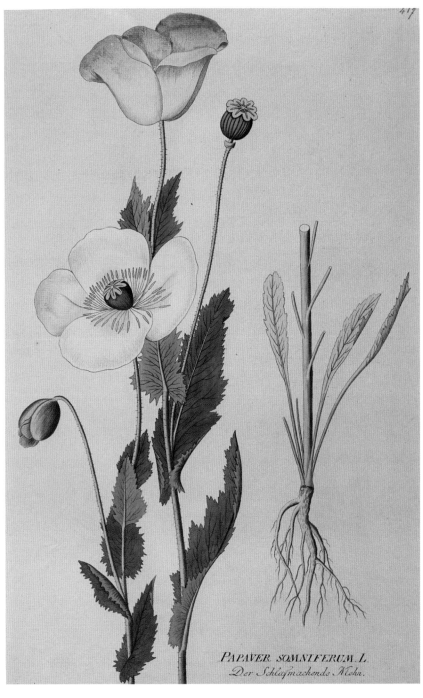

PAPAVER SOMNIFERUM. L.
Der Schlafmachende Mohn.

There are a number of diseases which can affect the opium plant and these usually have the effect of reducing crop yield. Fungal infections such as blight are the most common sources of disease but viruses and bacteria can also affect the whole plant or parts of it. Common pests that affect poppies are thrips, weevils and aphids, attacking the flowers, the pods and stems respectively.

Botanical illustration of opium poppies, from a nineteenth-century book of medicinal plants.

The method of harvesting opium has remained relatively unchanged for centuries. It can only be done by skilled manual labour and is particularly exhausting and labour-intensive. The harvest begins about a fortnight after the petals have dropped from the seed pod. The opium farmer first examines the pod and erect crown. By now, the pod will have lost its grey-green colour and darkened to a browner colour. If the points of the crown are standing straight out or curving upwards, the pod is ready. Not all the pods in a field will mature at the same time so the farmer has to maintain a daily regime on his whole crop over a period of some weeks. The instrument used for tapping the opium latex is usually a specialised knife and consists of three or four sharp parallel steel or glass edges mounted on a handle. When run over the sides of the pod, the opium starts to drip out. The cut has to be precise as if it is made too deeply then the pod will be damaged causing the whole plant to die back without seeding, having grave implications for not only this year's but next year's harvest too. If the cut is too shallow then the latex will not seep out sufficiently. Ideally, incisions should be made to a depth of 1–1.5mm or the plant may shrivel and die, preventing the seeds from developing, but if the cuts are too shallow, the outside of the pod may become hard and scab-like.

The opium starts out as a milky-white liquid, but on contact with the air it oxidises and turns into a dark brown molasses-like substance. It is scraped from the pod with a blunt iron blade and collected in containers. The farmers who work on licensed pharmaceutical farms clean the blades in water, whereas peasant farmers simply lick the blade, which often results in them becoming addicted to their crop. The pod continues to yield opium for several days and can be tapped several more times. The raw opium gum is then sundried for several days until it has reduced to a sticky gluelike substance. It is then beaten and kneaded and shaped into cakes or balls wrapped in plastic or leaves and stored in the shade.

As long as conditions are good, the opium will dry out, and become more concentrated. The raw opium is not pure, however. It may contain scrapes of the outer pod or other plant or even insect matter. In order to be refined it has to be cooked. This is done by adding the raw opium to boiling water in which it dissolves, leaving any impurities to rise to the surface of the water. It is then passed through cheesecloth or a fine sieve to remove impurities then brought to the boil again and reduced until all that remains is the clean brown liquid opium. When left to simmer it soon becomes a thick, brown paste known as prepared, cooked or smoking opium, which is pressed or moulded into trays and ready for use.

Freshly arrived liquid opium is weighed before being poured into trays to dry in the sunlight at a factory in Ghazipur.

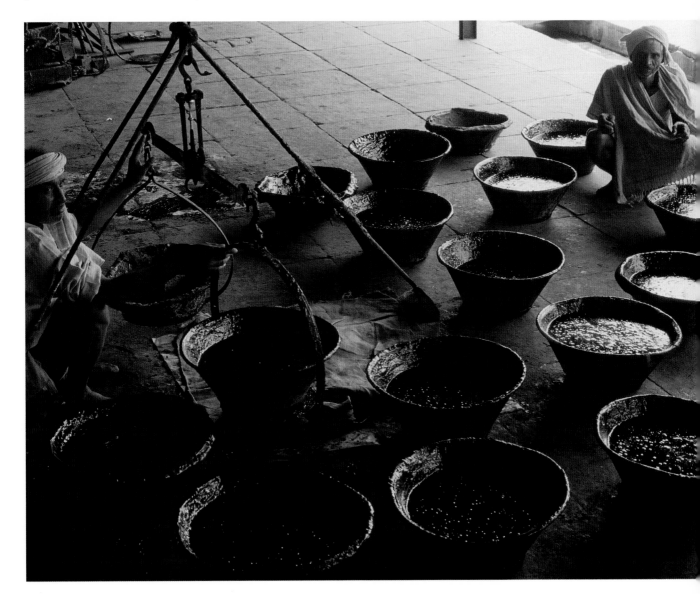

The drying trays have to be stired three times a day to prevent the opium from crusting.

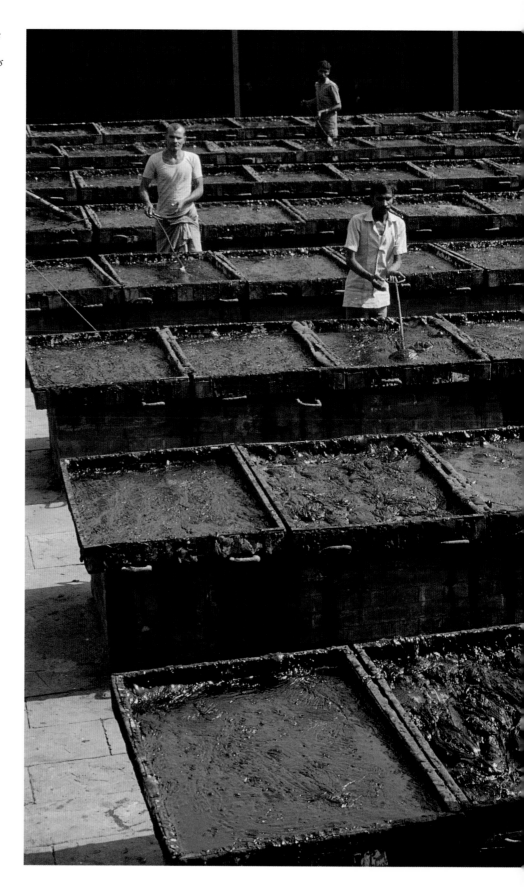

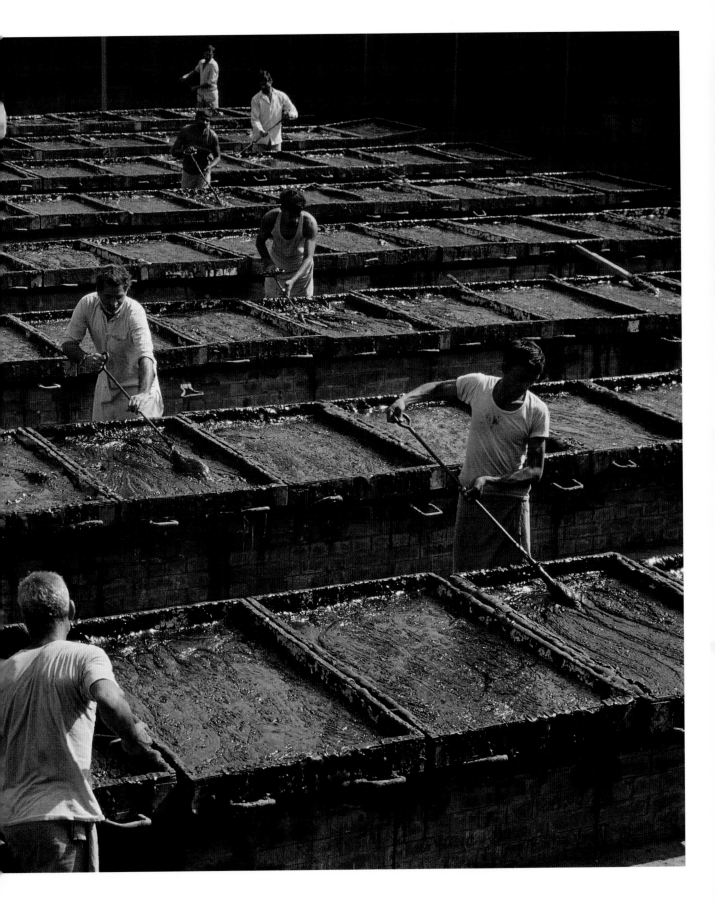

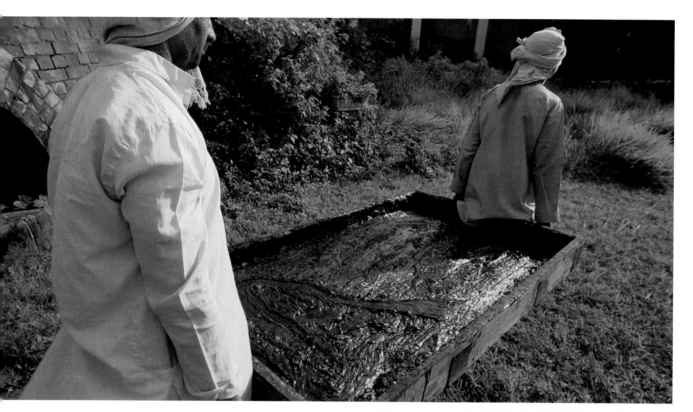

Opium being carried out to dry. The opium is reduce in the sunlight and concentrated down to 90% pure.

Historically, each area packaged its opium differently: Turkey produced 'Constantinople pats' which were small cakes wrapped in poppy leaves; Persia produced 'Trebizond', incense-like sticks; China produced 'Yunnan', cakes wrapped in white paper; and India produced 'Chandu' whereby it was rolled into small balls and covered with a layer of powdered leaves, capsules and stems. Often other spices were added to give different flavours.

The rest of the plant does not go to waste. Poppy straw, that is the stem and the poppy heads, can also been infused to create a sedative drink. However, it is illegal to possess poppy straw in many countries. The seeds once ripe are not dangerous and are used in cooking as decoration or as thickening agents. Many European countries utilise poppy seeds and ground seeds made into flour in their traditional cooking. The oil of the poppy seed is a rich source of linolic, oleic, palmitic and stearic acids. It can be used in cooking but has also been used in the manufacture of perfumes, as a base for artists' oil paints, and as lamp oil.

In India thousands of small landowners are licensed to grow opium, the production of which is controlled by the Central Narcotics Bureau which is a branch of India's Ministry of Finance. In the remote interiors of Northern India, acres of poppy fields produce tonnes of legal opium each year. Every year agricultural families are given licenses to grow opium poppies on 1/10 of a hectare on their small landholdings, on the condition that they harvest a minimum of 4.5kg (9.9lbs) of pharmaceutical-grade opium paste per year. Much of the land has been held by the same family for generations since the Moghul Empires. In India opium has always been used as a traditional medicine to cure diarrhoea and cure colicky babies but in modern times the opium is sold to pharmaceutical companies on an international basis.

Each year around 1,400 tonnes (1,378 tons) of opium are collected from these small farmers and shipped to one of two huge processing plants in Ghazipur in Uttar Pradesh and Nemuch in Madhya Pradesh. In these factories hundreds of workers attend row-upon-row of open air vats filled with black opium paste. Each vat can contain up to 65 tonnes (64 tons) of opium. For weeks on end the workers stir and turn this tar-like substance. It is then dried in the hot sun, each of the drying vats containing 40 tonnes (39 tons) of opium, until it loses most of its moisture. Once the opium has lost 90% of its moisture content it is repacked and is ready for sale. Most of this opium is exported to the USA, the UK, France and Japan and generates approximately £6 million in income per annum but the Indian pharmaceutical industry also retains some of the product for its own use. Without the legal opium industry many of these small farmers would struggle to make ends meet, since their landholdings are too small to raise sufficient cash crops. For each kilogram the farmer produces, he is paid the equivalent of £5, a fraction of the drug's value on the illegal market. The 4.5kg (9.9lbs) of opium that the Indian

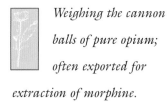

Weighing the cannon balls of pure opium; often exported for extraction of morphine.

farmer produces could produce 450g (15oz) of heroin which would have a street value of £50 per gramme, that is over £20,000. It is unsurprising to note that many of the farmers retain a portion of their harvest in order to sell into the illicit trade.

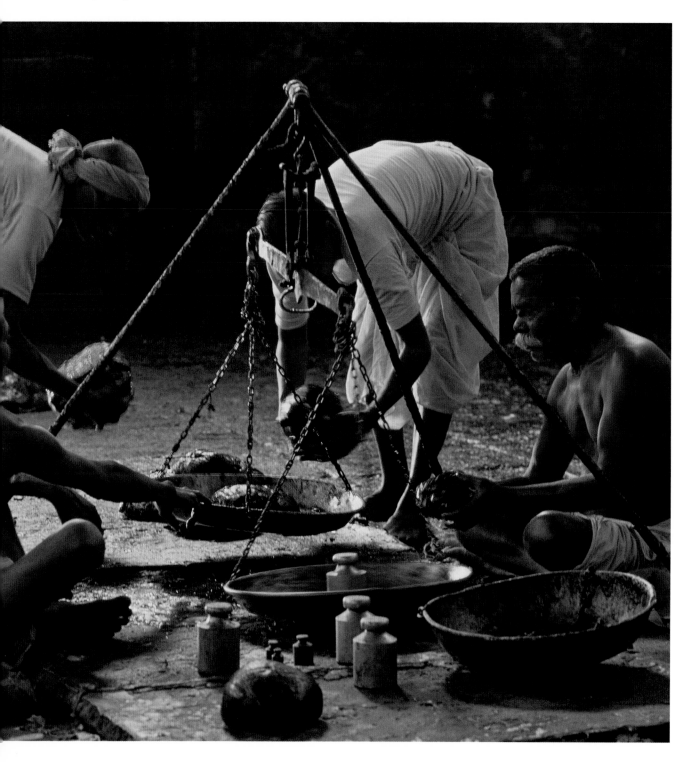

*'A man who would use opium for every little trivial ache
and pain would take an 80-ton gun to go rabbit shooting'*

A family physician c. 1900

*'Among the remedies which it has pleased Almighty God to
give to man to relieve his sufferings, none is so universal
and so efficacious as opium.'*

Thomas Sydenham (1624–89)

Opium has been used as a medicine for over 6,000 years but today only a very small quantity of opiates are used medicinally and indeed the UK is the only country in the world whose doctors are licensed to prescribe them as analgesics, particularly for patients suffering from terminal cancer, although in recent years this has become less prevalent. In medicine, the role of opium cannot be underestimated, its main medicinal use being obtained from its alkaloids and derivatives. It is the singularly most important painkiller available in the world.

*'I took possession of the throne and the royal realm and
rule the Kingdom justly. Let there be done production and
business dealing on toddy liquor, spirit, wine, beer, opium
and other narcotic substances in all the cities, towns and
villages of the realm and also in the Shan State and Yun
State (parts of present day Thailand and Laos). Illegal
animal slaughtering, husbandry, and gambling of all sorts
are prohibited and offenders will be punished severely'.*

King Badon (1782–1819)

A little girl holds a small dog on an advertising card for Dr. Seth Arnold's Cough Killer which sold for twenty-five cents. The product contained morphine.

The above passage is from the royal edict issued on 12 February 1728, the day when King Badon officially took possession of the throne. He was keen to collect ancient books on medicine, medicinal herbs and plants for use in various situations both as home remedies and for use on the battlefield. In the *Warhara Linathta Dipani*, a famous Myanmar encyclopaedia, it was stated that 'During the reign of the Lord of Amarapura (King Badon) the king showed the Bein and Bin plants to the Sinhalese monks from Ceylon, and queried about those flora. They explained to him that Bein was called "Ah-hi Phela" and Bin "Binga"'. Originally, bein (opium) was used as one of the ingredients in certain medicines and it was found in one of the royal edicts that King Badon allowed every soldier in the royal army to carry one measure of opium in the battlefield to prevent against disease and for use as a medicine and painkiller.

The dosing of infants with opium-based products and patent medicines during the nineteenth century was widespread and attracted much attention. Numerous 'soothing syrups' were on the open market in the Victorian Age, the most famous being Godfrey's Cordial, Street's Infants' Quietness, Atkinson's Infants' Preservative, and Mrs Winslow's, with many others made at home. The supply of these opium-based tinctures which were reputedly effective against colic, ensured that infants were added to the lists of opium dependants. In the 1840s Midland towns like Dudley and

TRY DR. SETH ARNOLD'S COUGH KILLER.

IT WORKS LIKE MAGIC Price 25 Cents.

OVER.

Sedgeley claimed sales of 70,000 bottles per year. This would explain the widespread use of laudanum amongst adults of this time; after having been given doses as children they became addicted and it became part of everyday life as much as aspirin is today.

> 'About all the field surgeon could do was use the two new invented tools that had been presented to him in the previous five or six years ... the hypodermic needle and syringe, along with Morphine Sulfate ... They injected the young wounded veterans with huge amounts of Morphine daily (every four hours) to kill their pain ... It was necessary for the surgeons to do full-quarter amputations — literally take the arms and legs off right at the start of the body, usually to stop infectious gangrene.'

(Mandel, J. (Date Unknown). *The Mythical Roots of US Drug Policy: Soldier's Disease and Addicts In The Civil War***. Quote from the work of Gerald Starkey)**

Opium and morphine were major painkillers and surgical anaesthetics used during the American Civil War (1861–5). Many wounded soldiers were sent home with them for pain relief. By the end of the war, over 400,000 people had what was known as the 'army disease', in other words, serious morphine addiction. The Franco-Prussian War in Europe had a similarly sad aftermath. In 1853 Dr Alexander Wood invented the hypodermic syringe based on designs by Sir Christopher Wren. He first used it to inject a dose of morphine. The previous method of injecting was with sharpened quills, a method used by Florence Nightingale herself. It was believed at the time that it was the smoking of opium that caused addiction and so the needle would reduce morphine addiction if the substance was injected directly into the bloodstream. Unfortunately, the result was that because

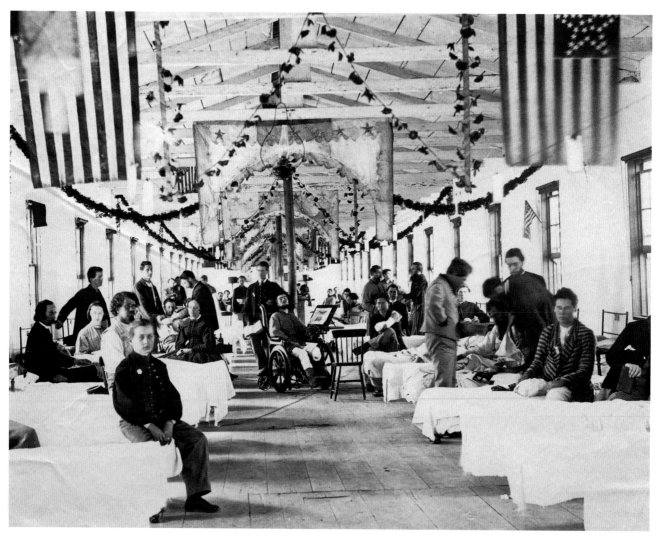

 View inside a ward of
the Armory Square
Hospital in
Washington, D.C., during
the American Civil War.

morphine works faster and is more effective when injected this way, more and more addicts were created.

'... The returning veteran could be identified because he had a leather thong around his neck and a leather bag [with] Morphine Sulfate tablets, along with a syringe and a needle issued to the soldier on his discharge ... [T]his was called the 'Soldier's Disease.'

Gerald Starkey

Opium poppies contain up to 50 alkaloids (alkaloid was the name given to salt-forming organic alkali by Wilheim Meissner in 1818). Of these, morphine and codeine are the most well-known.

Morphine

Although the first use of morphine can be traced to 4000 BC, it was not until 1803 when Jean-François Derosne, a Parisian pharmacist, isolated crystalline morphine from opium, that the drug became famous. Later experiments by Wilhelm Sertürner on dogs, showed that when the morphine was mixed with the dogs' weaning milk, the effects were narcotic. This discovery was largely ignored until it was translated into French and taken up by Gay-Lussac, who heralded the idea that Morphine was a new group of salt-forming alkali. In 1925 J.M Gulland and R. Robinson found the correct chemical structure for morphine. 7,8-didehydro-4,5-epoxy-17-methyl(5alpha,6alpha)-morphinan-3,6-diol or $C_{17}H_{19}O_3N$.

Morphine was praised by physicians and trumpeted as 'God's own medicine' for its safety, positive effects and overall effectiveness. Morphine has analgesic properties, which can alleviate feelings of pain without the subject losing consciousness, although it can make them drowsy. Unfortunately, it is highly addictive. After heroin, morphine has the greatest dependence liability of all the narcotic analgesics. It can be administered via several routes – injected, sniffed, swallowed or smoked. When injected morphine produces intense euphoria and a general state of wellbeing and relaxation, no matter how severe the physical pain that a patient is enduring. Unfortunately, regular use results in the rapid development of tolerance and for the need to increase dosage. Owing to the euphoric state of being that the drug induces, profound psychological dependence also develops on a rapid basis.

Early Bayer Pharmaceutical Advertisement. Bayer introduced heroin in 1898 as a cough suppressant that did not have the harmful effects of other opiates. Aspirin was produced in the same Bayer laboratories and released to the public a year later.

Morphine is produced under the licensed names Roxinal and Morphine Sulphate. On the street it is more commonly known as 'Miss Emma' or 'M' or 'Morph' and is a Class A drug. It is legally available in the UK in the form of its water-soluble salts called morphine hydrochloride and morphine sulphate, both of which are white crystalline powders with a bitter taste. Kaolin morphine, a mixture of clay and morphine, is available as an over-the-counter medication for stomach upsets. The optimal intramuscular dosage is 10mg per 70kg (154lbs) of bodyweight every four hours. Illegal users have been known to take up to 4,000mg per day.

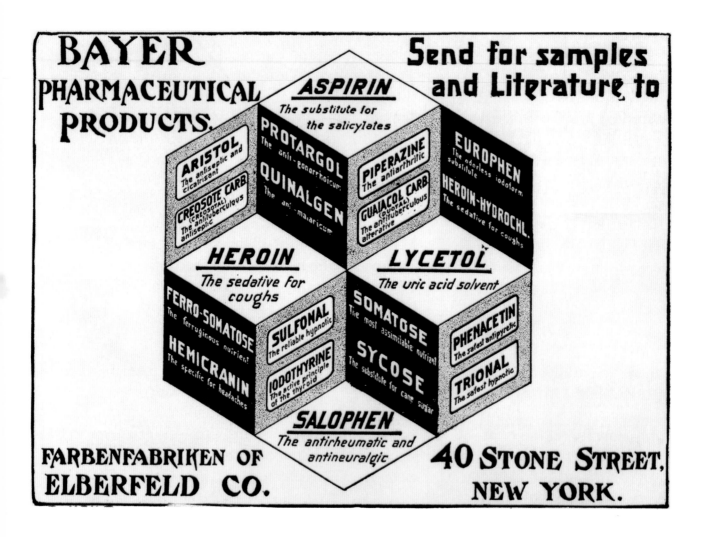

80

Codeine

Codeine is found in opium in concentrations of between 1–2%. Owing to the small concentrations, most medical codeine is synthesised from morphine. Its street name is '3Ts', 'Schoolboy' or 'Cough Syrup'. Codeine is usually prescribed as a cough treatment, as a mild analgesic and for diarrhoea and is nearly always taken orally. A 30mg dose will mimic the effects of morphine except sedation and euphoria are less intense. Codeine is a Class B drug unless for medicinal purposes.

Heroin

In 1898 Heinrich Dreser of the Friedrich Bayer and Company first introduced Heroin (medical name of diamorphine) to the world. This was named after the word 'heroic', due to its energising and stimulating effect. It was thought to be a safer version of morphine, containing diacetylmorphine (acetylated morphine with the chemical formula $C_{17}H_{17}NO(C_2H_3O_2)_2$) thought to be a new wonder-drug. The manufacture of heroin involves many processes: first equal quantities of morphine and acetic anhydride are heated in a glass container for 6 hours, the morphine and the acid combining to form impure diacetyle-morphine, next water and chloroform are added to precipitate any impurities, the solution is then drained and sodium carbonate is added to make the heroin solidify and sink; the heroin is then filtered out using activated charcoal and then purified with alcohol. The remaining solution is then evaporated to remove the alcohol and so leave the heroin which may be purified further or converted to heroin hydrochloride, a water-soluble heroin salt. It became phenomenally popular. Hailed ironically as a cure for opium addiction, it could even be purchased by mail order through the Sears Catalogue. With as many as 1,000,000 addicts in America alone by 1900, it was becoming clear that this 'heroic' drug as it was romantically called, was actually becoming frighteningly dangerous.

Opposite: A hypodermic syringe containing heroin

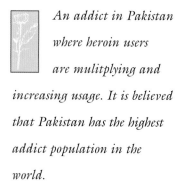

An addict in Pakistan where heroin users are mulitplying and increasing usage. It is believed that Pakistan has the highest addict population in the world.

Not surprising when you realise that heroin is four times as potent as morphine and is metabolised by the body at twice the rate: in effect, this miracle drug was no more than another insidiously destructive version of the opiate. It has a very high rate of physical dependency and as we now know is one of the most addictive drugs to ever be created.

Although heroin comes into the country up to 90% pure, it is then diluted using milk powder or lactose, the act being called 'cutting'. Many deaths these days are caused by addicts overdosing on product that has not been cut as much as they are used to. The Colombians particularly pride themselves on the quality of their new product which unfortunately is too pure.

The major problem with modern heroin use is the 'high' reduces as tolerance rises and addicts end up taking the drug just to feel normal. The original euphoria becomes increasingly difficult to achieve and then is lost completely. By this stage physical dependency is firmly established and so most addicts increase their doses in order to try to regain it and begin taking drug cocktails such as 'speedballs' (heroin with cocaine), 'uppers' (amphetamines), 'downers' (barbituates) or methedrine.

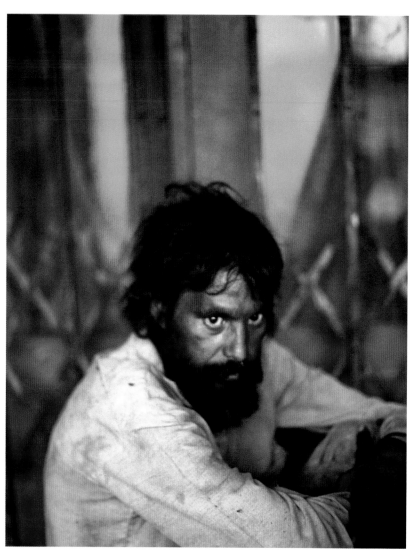

Opioids

A number of synthetic opiums called opioids are also manufactured today for medical use. These include dihydrocodeine (DF118), pethidine which is often used to alleviate pain in childbirth, dichonal, palfium, temgesic and physeptone. Opiods are compounds which possess an affinity for the opioid receptor subtypes in the brain. They are not structured in the same way as morphine but have similar properties and effects. The most common known ones are endorphins which are naturally-produced painkillers in the human body and the synthetic Methadone, which is the substitute used to wean addicts from heroin. Methadone was invented by the Germans during the Second World War as a field painkiller for soldiers. It has less euphoric qualities than heroin and so was used in clinical trials as another replacement therapy for heroin addicts. It can be prescribed by doctors for registered addicts. Unfortunately, it has since been found that it is as addictive as heroin itself. Another recently developed semi-synthetic opiate is called etorphine, also known as M99 or immobilon is 10,000 times as powerful as morphine with less than 2ml able to render a full-grown rhinoceros senseless.

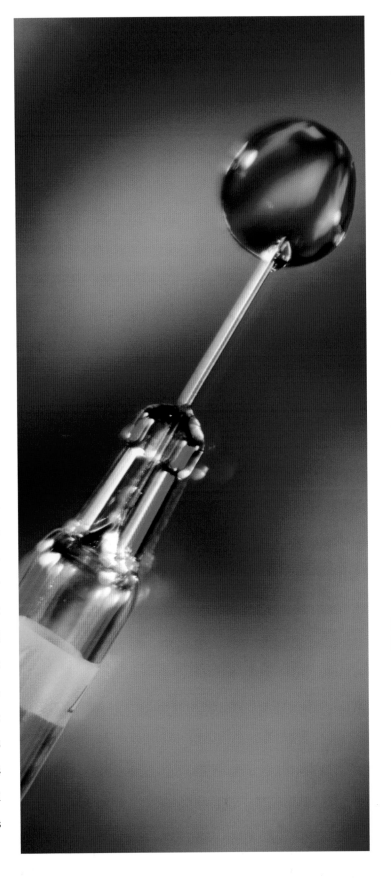

The pharmacological effects of opiates result from the fact that these substances have a bit (like a key) just like the endorphins and thus directly stimulate the endorphin receptors in the body because they latch on in the same way. Because the opiates were known earlier than the endorphins the neuroanatomists named them opiate receptors. The receptors in the brain can be traced by injecting radioactive opiates and then monitoring where the radioactivity collects in the brain. This appears to be in very specific areas. The first concentration of opiate receptors is formed by a nerve cell system which plays a vital role in the transmission of pain stimuli. For example, if you prick yourself on a needle the first impulse is to put the bleeding finger in the mouth before any pain is felt. This is because a reflex is sent via the spinal cord and immediately returned to the arm muscles. This route is extremely fast. At the same time the message is transmitted to the cortex of the cerebrum which results in the first experience of pain by going to the higher centres of the brain. Until then there are only signals aimed at a direct reaction to end the pain. However, in order to prevent this happening again, every time the finger is injured, a moment of learning is sent slowly from the spinal cord to the part of the brain stem where the opiate receptors are located. This area is responsible for the alarming or threatening aspect of pain and it is exactly this effect which is remedied so effectively by the taking of opiates.

The feeling of pain itself does not disappear but it loses the threatening character and in effect the pain starts to become less noticeable. The most striking quality of this painkilling effect of opiates is that it has virtually no effect whatsoever on the other sensory perceptions, i.e. consciousness or the motor functions. All other substances with a painkilling effect such as laughing gas, ether, alcohol and barbiturates also have a definite effect on consciousness, motor co-ordination, the intellect and emotional control. The drowsiness that can be caused by opiates is only experienced at very high dosage.

A concentration of opiate receptors are also located in the respiratory centre of the brain and serve as a kind of metronome by regulating the breath. Opiates also have an inhibiting effect on these cells. Both the frequency and depth of breathing is reduced under the effect of opiates, so much so that in the case of an overdose, respiration can cease altogether. Opiates also inhibit sensitivity of the impulse to cough by again affecting the reflex pathway. The third concentration is in the vomiting centre of the brain which when stimulated by the stomach normally causes the stomach muscles to contract, resulting in vomiting. These cells are stimulated into activity by opiates. Opiate use therefore can cause nausea and vomiting but tolerance is built up very rapidly. This effect is strongest with the

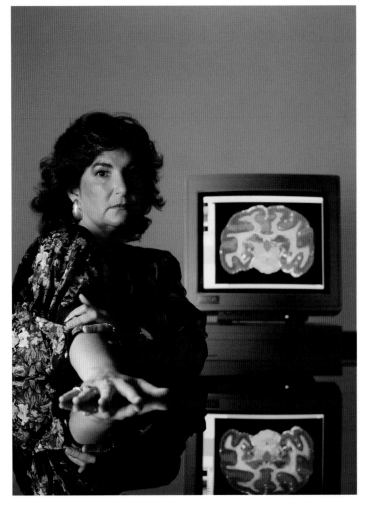

opiate called apomorphine which is used medically specifically for this purpose. The effect of opiates on the digestive system, which also contains large numbers of receptors, has been known for the longest period of time. Long before opiates were used as painkillers they were used to relieve the symptoms of diarrhoea due to its ability to inhibit intestinal contractions. It is for this reason that most heroin addicts are constipated. Opiates also affect the endocrine system, that is, the hormonal and glandular system. By affecting the hypothalamus body temperature is slightly lowered which results in addicts often being cold until they get to a high level of addiction whereby they get the 'sweats'. Opiates also lower the amount of cortisol and testosterone in the blood, resulting in lethargy and a lowered sexual drive although again these effects disappear with chronic use.

Portrait of neurologist and author Candice Pert sitting by a CAT scan on a monitor. Pert is credited with the discovery of the opiate receptor and is a pioneer in the field of emotions.

Opiates contract the pupils which is one of the most reliable indicators of opiate useage. In the case of an overdose the pupils dilate. In the usual therapeutic dosage morphine widens the veins in the skin, giving a flushed appearance and a warm sensation. This is through the release of histamine that morphine induces and can result in itching and perspiration.

Addiction and Cure

'I've never had a problem with drugs. I've had problems with the police.'

Keith Richards

In the 1960s the World Health Organisation used 'dependence' to replace the terms addiction and habituation and defined it as 'a state, psychic and sometimes also physical resulting from the interaction between a living organism and a drug characterised by behavioural and other responses that always include a compulsion to take the drug on a continuous or periodic basis in order to experience its psychic effects and sometimes to avoid the discomfort of its absence. Tolerance may or may not be present.' This definition thus shows that drug dependence is both psychological and physical and also avoided making a negative value judgement on individual drug users.

The words 'kick' and 'rush' are bandied about amongst opiate dependents, specifically heroin users, as part of their street jargon. The effects of taking opiates are described as a warm sensation that spreads through the stomach and to the groin and that often results in an orgasmic feeling. This continues so that the addict perceives that they are in a safe, womb-like state of physical and emotional wellbeing. All pain ceases and the user is able to escape into a state of tranquillity as well as complete freedom from anxiety and stress, at least whilst the levels of opiates are above a certain threshold. As the levels decrease the state of being before using returns. Once dependence has been established, usually on a second dose, returning to a state of existence without opiates is impossible to bear. The addict must obtain opiates or they will become anxious and unable to cope with pain. A lack of drugs may even lead to death as the body and mind have become so used to the presence of opiates that a state of shock is entered.

By the end of the nineteenth century and onwards, a range of treatments and cures were sought for the opium curse. In the early 1900s Dr. Alexander Lambert and Charles B. Towns sold their cure, the Towns Treatment, as the most 'advanced, effective and compassionate cure' for opium addiction. The cure involved a seven-day regimen, which included a five-day purge of heroin from the addict's system with doses of belladonna delirium and digitalis. The withdrawal from addiction to opiates is commonly known as 'cold turkey' and involves the addict developing severe flu'-like symptoms – aches, tremors, sweating, chills and muscular spasms. They fade after 7–10 days but a feeling of weakness may persist. Whilst many people successfully give up long-term use, coming off and then staying off can be extremely difficult. Many addicts proselytise others and see addiction as entry into an elite club with its own cultural and linguistic rules. Also it is much easier to score and use in an area where there are plenty of addicts than being a single addict.

At present, there are various methods of treating opiate addiction. In the UK methadone is prescribed to addicts who register with the Drug Dependency Unit. Having done that, they are interviewed by a panel of six people, including psychologists and social workers and then in order to take their daily dose of methadone they must personally visit a local pharmacy and take the methadone in liquid form in front of the chemist. This ensures that the methadone does not end up on the black market. However, methadone itself is far more addictive than heroin and has longer withdrawal symptoms and, unlike heroin which only stays in the system for 72 hours, methadone stays in the system for months. This is a treatment reminiscent of the time when heroin was considered a treatment for morphine addiction.

Outside the National Health Service of the UK, opiate dependents who can afford it can travel to Spain where there is a 72-hour sleep cure clinic or travel to Switzerland for a three-week cure which includes sleep, therapy and a change of blood via transfusion. The Swiss cure is really only suitable for the rich and famous due to its high cost. In the USA, a drug called Disulfiram that is implanted subcutaneously on a monthly basis is often given to addicts. Its effect is to cause severe nausea and vomiting should the reformed addict attempt to ingest even the smallest dose of opiates. There are also the Narcotics Anonymous Programs across America which offer cure and rehabilitation to addicts. In the UK there are estimated to be just over 200,000 heroin abusers, many of whom are repeat offenders within the prison system. Sadly, at present, this rate of addiction is increasing by 20% per annum. New programmes and new ways of thinking about cure and rehabilitation are needed badly. Recently small-scale experiments have been introduced in the UK whereby addicts are prescribed heroin rather than methadone. Certainly, the people within these programmes have reported benefits in that they have been able to stop criminal aspects of their behaviour such as stealing and prostitution which they would normally use to fund their habit.

Opioids, unlike opiates, have specific withdrawal and dependence charac-teristics, depending on each specific drug. All cause both physical and psychological dependence, often in as short a time as a fortnight of use. Withdrawal itself, although commonly overstated in the media, tends like morphine to be no worse than a bad case of flu', although the psychological withdrawal can produce deep trauma. Depression, mood

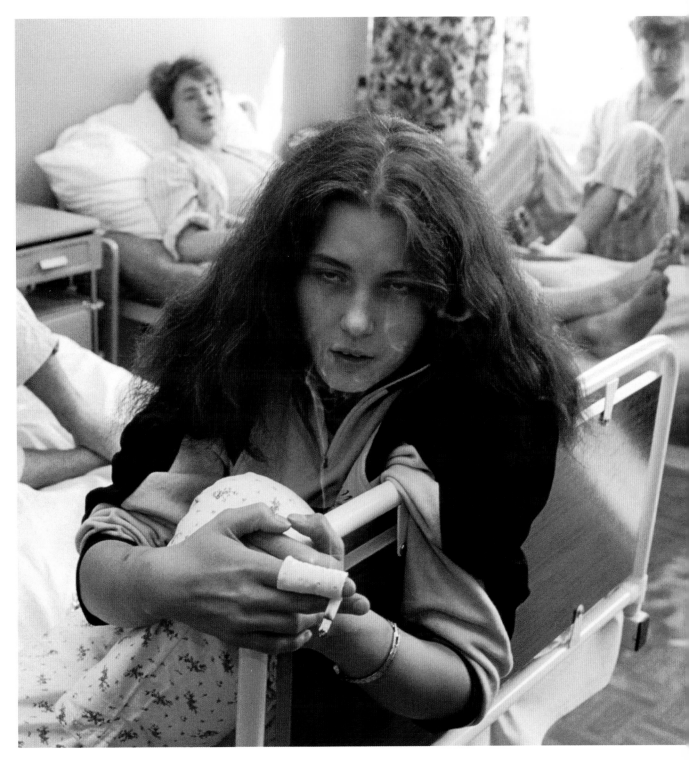

swings and hypersensitivity to pain all prevail, but opioid withdrawal does not endanger life and it could be argued that it is the criminal behaviour that addicts turn to in order to fund their habits that causes more problems to society at large than the addiction itself.

Patients in a temporary heroin detox clinic.

A detailed oil on silk image of a smoker and young divan hostesses.

'I've seen some things that people would call strange enough: but nothing is strange when you are on the Black Smoke, except the black smoke'

Rudyard Kipling (1865–1936)

The image of the opium den is often a lurid one. Generally the idealised version including soft Arabic cushions, incense and beautiful young things all lying around in various states of dreaming is a rarity. More often than not, an opium den is a dimly-lit room, sparsely furnished, with filthy cushions for the smoker to rest his head on whilst partaking of the pipe. Depending on the whereabouts of the room, the interior would have to be easily disguised in case of a swoop by the authorities. The room would have to be sealed well, so that no opium fumes could escape. Often in the more heavily populated and squalid rooms there would be wooden bunks furnished with small bundles of straw or papers for the smoker to use as a pillow, or sometimes a filthy mat to lie on would be all the furniture present. It was important for the opium addict to smoke in company, not because of any conversation that might take place, but purely for the comfort of having other souls near them. Although many images of opium smoking have sensual or erotic themes, in fact there is no connection to how the smoker feels. Even if aroused the effect of the drug is that to pacify, dull and dope down the senses, movement is lazy and the feeling is an insular one. The smoker is caught up in their own world, a dream that is theirs alone. Women who frequented opium dens added a sexual overtone to various writers' imaginative descriptions. Authors such as Arthur Conan Doyle in the Sherlock Holmes short story *The Twisted Lip*, Charles Dickens in *The Mystery of Edwin Drood*, Sax Rohmer in his Fu Manchu series, and Thomas Burke, whose famous story *The Chink and the Child* was made into a film in 1919 called 'Broken Blossoms', all successfully captivated the public with their lurid descriptions of opium den depravity and exoticism.

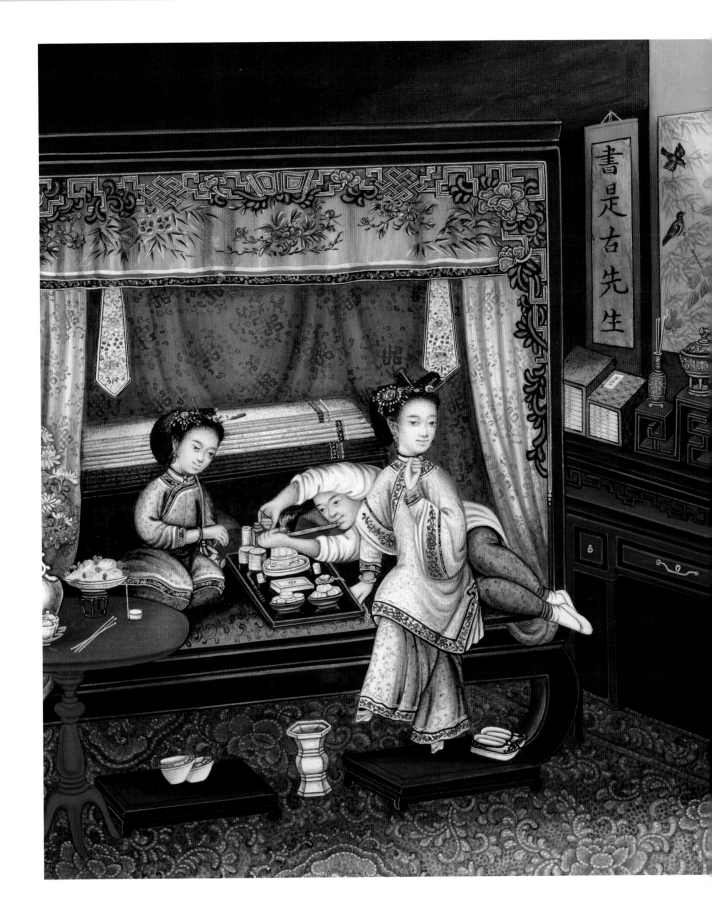

書是古先生

'Oh, wicked little dope pill,
You sphere of poppy dough –
Tho' sin to oft indulged in –
I fonder of you grow.

Thou dear, diverting hop pill,
That makes all care forgot;
Without you what would life be?
A drear and tasteless lot.

The Tenderloin girls all love you,
You are their heart's delight;
The sight of you brings sunshine;
Your absence – darkest night'

The Lay of a Lotus Eater by Louis J Becke (1859–1913)

A typical opium kit includes a pipe, a long needle or pin, a spirit lamp of some sort and a box of opium paste. These are usually presented on a tray. In well-to-do dens, there would be someone to prepare the pipes for those present and perhaps to make tea for them. The opium pipe is usually a 46–61cm (18–24in) long flute shape with a removable bowl with a small hole in the top attached for the opium to be placed inside. It is sealed at one end, with a mouthpiece at the other. The construction of the pipe is such that no smoke can escape apart from through the mouthpiece. The pipe must be kept horizontal with the bowl upright to avoid spillage, hence the images of opium smokers lying on their side to partake of the drug. Depending on the finances of the pipe owner, this could be an elaborate affair made in ebony, amber or ivory and covered with jewels and engravings and with a jade or amber mouthpiece, or it could be a simple wooden or bamboo construction. Bamboo however absorbs the fumes of the drug and become mellower over time. Opium smokers became very attached to their pipes, as the care of the pipe would have a direct effect on the quality of the smoke.

First the spirit lamp is lit, and the smoker takes a small pill of the opium paste and spears it with the needle. This is gently held over the flame of the lamp until the brown mass starts to bubble and cook. The smoker may allow the pill to catch fire, quickly blowing it out and stretching the opium so that it becomes molasses-like, stringy and warm. The opium is then rolled back into a small ball and pushed into the hole in the top of the pipe which is held close to the flame. The smoker then takes deep puffs on

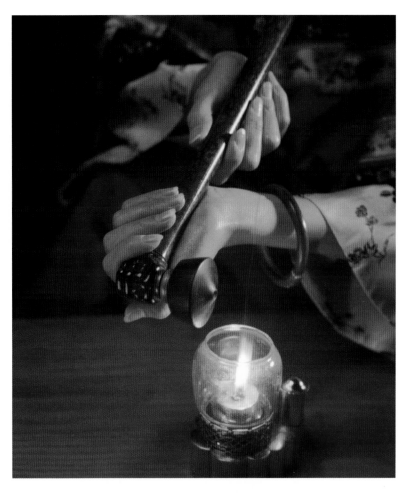

 A Chinese lady lovingly warming her bowl of opium.

the pipe and very soon the opium is gone with the effect being virtually instantaneous. The smoker must recline and let the effect take over, sometimes this requires a build-up. It was not uncommon for the seasoned smoker to consume several pipes before they feel satisfied. One piece of modern jargon that is bandied around without people realising that it is associated with opium. The word is 'hip', meaning to be part of the current scene although its original meaning comes from the nineteenth century when a 'hip' was an experienced drug taker because addicts gained sore hips from reclining on their sides on the hard boards in opium dens. The history of opium is also part of the history of the arts: warriors, politicians, musicians, painters, writers and mystics ... from Roman generals to Romantic poets and rock icons, many have succumbed to opium and its beguiling charms. It is muse to many and a nightmare to others.

OPIUM AND LEADERSHIP

When Alexander the Great introduced opium to the Indians and Persians in 330 BC was he was already one of the greatest military figures in history. He conquered much of what was then the civilised world, driven by an intense ambition to create a universal world monarchy.

This romantic figure is described as being a strong, handsome man, apparently one eye was as dark as the night and one blue as a cloudless summer sky. He conquered Greece, Egypt, Asia Minor, and Asia up to western India and was famous for having created the ethnic fusion of the Macedonians and the Persians. Known to ride a beautiful horse called Bucephalus, he was the first great conqueror. Through a succession of military victories, Alexander created an empire which ensured him fame and fortune. He introduced Greek ideas, culture and lifestyle to the countries where he travelled, and assured the steady expansion and domination of Hellenistic Culture which, together with Roman Civilisation and Christianity, constitutes the foundation of what is now called Western Civilisation. He also seemed to be a fan of the opium plant, and reputedly introduced it to many cultures including Persia and India.

A detail of a mosaic from Naples, Italy. It depicts a battle between Alexander the Great and Darius III, King of Persia.

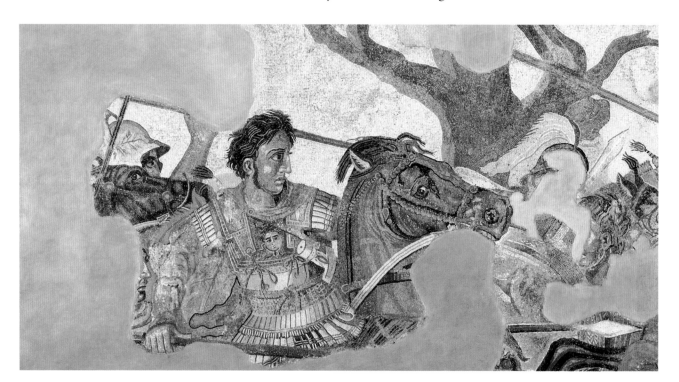

'At dawn of day, when you dislike being called, have this thought ready: "I am called to man's labour; why then do I make a difficulty if I am going out to do what I was born to do and what I was brought into the world for?"'

Marcus Aurelius (AD 121–180)

Marcus Aurelius, the legendary Roman leader, was the only emperor whose life was devoted to philosophy. He was born into a distinguished family, and grew up at one of the most peaceful times in the history of the Roman Empire. As a child, he won many public prizes for both rhetoric and philosophy, and it seems that even as young as eight years old, he was marked out as successor by the Emperor Hadrian. By the time Marcus turned 40, he was a deeply committed stoic, believing strongly in the power of reason to override life's tragedies. He was also an opium addict. Legend has it opium was initially prescribed to him because he suffered terrible joint pains but Marcus was a depressive personality, ill-suited to the military role his leadership thrust upon him, and more interested in universal philosophy and the soul than affairs of state. He quickly became addicted. Marcus spent the last few years of his life fighting the barbarians on the northern frontier. He died of a mystery illness, and his son, Commodus (reputed to have secured the 'decline and fall' of the Roman Empire) succeeded him.

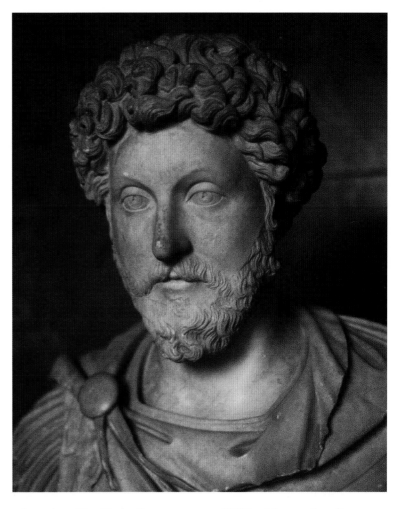

Marcus Aurelius.

'... little remains of me but a skeleton covered with a skin.'

Benjamin Franklin (1706–90)

Benjamin Franklin by Joseph Siffred Duplessis, 1783. North Carolina Museum of Art.

Benjamin Franklin, printer and publisher, author, inventor and scientist and diplomat, was probably the most famous eighteenth century American next to George Washington. A perfect example of the American dream, Franklin was born the tenth of seventeen children of a soap and candlemaker, and ended his formal education at the age of 10. But tenaciously he taught himself to write, and by 1757 had made a small fortune with his 'Poor Richard' Almanacs (an oracle on how to get ahead in the world) and was renowned world-wide for his experiments with electricity and his invention of the stove (which is still being manufactured today). This was only the beginning of his long and distinguished career in politics. In 1775 Franklin returned to America from his petitioning in England, fearing imminent war. He was immediately drafted into the Second Continental Congress, and helped compose the Declaration of Independence. In the same year Franklin went to Paris to negotiate financial and military support from the revolutionaries there. He was hailed as a hero and his face was everywhere, from snuff-boxes to chamber pots but whilst in Paris, Franklin became excruciatingly ill with a stone in his bladder. He began to take opium to subdue the pain, although he was terrified by its hallucinatory powers. He returned to America, unable to walk and bedridden. He began writing his autobiography (mostly under the influence of opium), but was unable to complete it. He died an opium addict.

'Look upon me, O Lord, with compassion and mercy, and restore me to rest, quietness, and comfort in the world, or in another by removing me hence into a state of happiness.'

William Wilberforce (1759–1833)

William Wilberforce was born into a wealthy Devonshire family. He was a very sickly child, blighted by weak and painful eyes that would sometimes turn to sacks of blood, and a stomach prone to colic. He was given opium as a pain-reliever and a cure for colitis, but he was unhappy taking it – he found the depressions were crippling. For many years, his body had to be held upright by a crude metal frame, and his doctor gloomily reported 'That little fellow, with his calico guts, cannot possibly survive a twelve-month.' He did, but in the process became heavily dependent on opium. He studied at Cambridge, where he

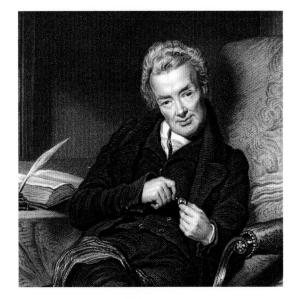

William Wilberforce.

became a close friend of the future Prime Minister William Pitt the Younger. In 1780 both he and Pitt entered the House of Commons, and Wilberforce quickly acquired a reputation for radicalism due to his support of parliamentary reform and Roman Catholic political emancipation. In 1787, inspired by his Evangelical beliefs, Wilberforce helped found a society for the Abolition of the Slave Trade. Dedicated and tireless, Wilberforce agitated, petitioned and argued until, in 1807, he achieved his first success – a bill was passed that abolished the slave trade in the British West Indies. Now it was time to have slavery wiped out entirely: despite his increasingly bad health, Wilberforce continued work and became president of the Society for the Mitigation and Gradual Abolition of Slavery Throughout the British Dominions. He died one month before the Slavery Abolition Act he had dreamed of was passed in the House of Commons.

'Can't you see, Sister Morphine, I'm just trying to score.
Well, it just goes to show things are not what they seem.
Please, Sister Morphine, turn my nightmare into dreams.
Oh, can't you see I'm fading fast
And that this shot will be my last.
Sweet Cousin Cocaine, lay your cool hands on my head.
Hey, Sister Morphine, you'd better make up my bed
For you know and I know in the morning I'll be dead,
And you can sit around and you can watch the clean white
sheets stain red.'

Sister Morphine by Keith Richards
and Mick Jagger.
From the album Sticky Fingers (1971).

Since the days when opium dens ceased to function and with the advent of modern derivatives such as heroin and morphine, the user has become more recreational than medicinal. On the street opiates, in particular heroin, have been given their own language. To 'shoot up' or 'mainline' is to inject intravenously and the equipment used to inject is called 'artillery'. To 'chase the dragon' or 'tiger' is to smoke it. Heroin itself is called by such slang terms as 'China Red', 'China White', 'candy', 'Horse', 'H', 'Big Harry', 'Mexican Mud', 'elephant', 'skag', 'sweet stuff', 'gear', 'junk', 'smack' and 'brown sugar', the latter famously immortalised in the Rolling Stones' song of the same name. As the heroin works the user 'nods off'. To be addicted is to have 'a monkey on your back' or be 'strung out', a dealer is a 'juggler' (usually someone who uses as well) a 'pusher', 'candyman', 'connection' or 'the man'. Heroin is sold by the 'spoon' ($\frac{1}{16}$th of an ounce), 'the deal', 'the deck', the 'piece', the 'half-lo' and the 'key' (one kilogram) all of which refer to the quantity.

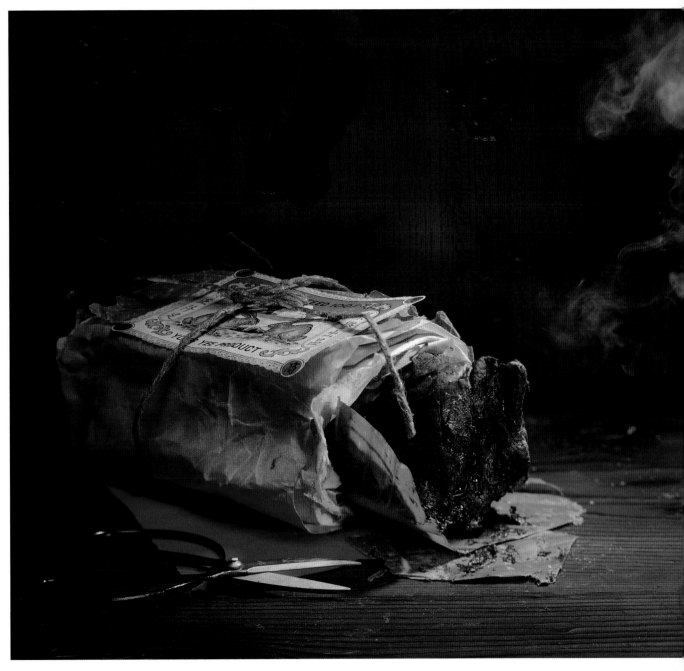

The culture which has evolved around opium has heavily influenced many of our musicians, either through song lyrics or through their lifestyles. Keith Richards of the Rolling Stones had a well-documented battle with heroin addiction and as previously mentioned, many of the Stones' songs feature it heavily in their lyrics.

Opium wrapped in it protective covering of banana leaf.

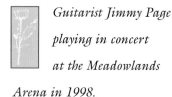

Guitarist Jimmy Page playing in concert at the Meadowlands Arena in 1998.

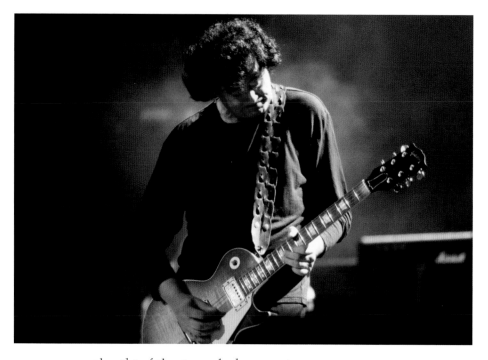

'Oh, pilot of the storm who leaves no trace
Like thoughts inside a dream
Heed the path that led me to that place
Yellow desert screen
My Shangri-La beneath the summer moon
I will return again
As the dust that floats high in June
When movin' through Kashmir'

**Kashmir by Jimmy Page, Robert Plant
and John Bonham (Led Zeppelin).
From the album Physical Graffiti (1975).**

Led Zeppelin wrote the song *Kashmir*, once one of the prime areas for opium poppy growth, and although there is no evidence to suggest that any members of the band were personally takers of opium derivatives, the guitarist Jimmy Page was known to be an avid collector of Aleister Crowley first editions and lived in Crowley's house, Boleskine, on the shores of Loch Ness.

100

"Cause when the smack begins to flow
Then I really don't care anymore
Ah, when the heroin is in my blood
And that blood is in my head
Then thank God that I'm as good as dead
Then thank your God that I'm not aware
And thank God that I just don't care
And I guess I just don't know'

Heroin by Lou Reed (1967)

Another famous musician/songwriter who had a battle with the demon of heroin is Lou Reed. He wrote the immortal song *Heroin* which is full of slang terminology for the drug.

'I'll die before I'm 25, and when I do I'll have lived
the way I wanted to.'

Sid Vicious (1958–78)

Probably the most famous drug casualty of modern times was Sid Vicious. John Simon Ritchie was born in May 1958, the only child of a single parent in London's East End. He was growing up amongst claustrophobic estate blocks and bored drug-users when he met the infamous John Lydon (Johnny Rotten). Rotten had formed a band called the Sex Pistols, and by 1976 their anarchic lyrics and thrashing chords had broken the headlines. Now calling himself 'Sid Vicious' he used to go along to the gigs. Angry, violent, and in love with Punk, Vicious quickly replaced the original bassist, and aged just 18, was catapulted into rock'n'roll stardom. The band attracted notoriety and fame and would constantly be in the British music press. Around the same time a disaffected 20-year-old groupie named Nancy Spungen arrived in London from New York.

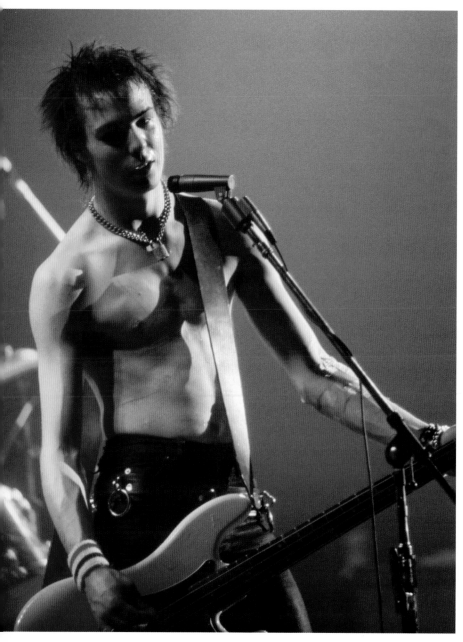

*Sid Vicious of
the Sex Pistols*

Spungen had a history of drug abuse, and in particular heroin. She quickly became involved with Sid. They had a strangled, year-long relationship, during which time Nancy introduced Sid to heroin. By 1978, Sid Vicious was a full-blown heroin addict, aged 20. He suffered from terrible fits of depression, and unable to see anything outside of his miserable and painful mood swings, as well as those of Nancy, he started on a downward spiral. The couple would argue constantly; it seemed that Sid felt that nothing was working in his head or in his life. Later that year, the receptionist at the Chelsea Hotel in New York where the couple were staying received a call for help: Nancy Spungen had been found dead under the sink, in a pool of her own blood, and Vicious was lying in bed virtually comatose. Ten days later he was freed on bail, a plethora of conspiracy theories surrounding Spungen's death. That evening, Vicious found a broken lightbulb and disposable razor in his hotel room and slashed his wrists, but did not die. Whether or not Vicious had accidentally killed Nancy with a knife in a fit of heroin-withdrawal we will never know. However his moods became blacker and blacker and eventually two months later, Vicious overdosed on heroin. He was only 21 years old.

'Not poppy, not mandragore,

Nor all the drowsy syrups in the world,

Shall ever medicine thee to that sweet sleep

which thou owedst Yesterday'

Act III, Scene 3 of *Othello*

'Weave a circle round him thrice,

And close your eyes with holy dread,

For he on honey-dew hath fed,

And drunk the milk of Paradise.'

Kubla Khan by Samuel Taylor Coleridge (1772–1834)

Samuel Taylor Coleridge was born in Ottery St. Mary in 1772, the youngest of the ten children of John Coleridge, a minister and teacher. He was a sickly child, and was prescribed laudanum as a pain-reliever. Nevertheless, he was a prodigy, and devoured books such as The Arabian Nights. He won a place to study at Jesus College, Cambridge, and it was here he discovered the visionary potential of opium and that it kept the depressions and anxieties at bay. He became heavily addicted, and carried a silver bottle of laudanum around his neck for the rest of his life. In 1794, he dropped out of Cambridge in a fit of revolutionary fervour, to lead anarchist uprisings in Bristol. There he met fellow poet Wordsworth and together they moved to Nether Stowey, Somerset. Poets, painters and political activists visited the house, and the two men lived in a haze of bohemian bliss. It was at Nether Stowey that Coleridge wrote the brilliant dream-like and visionary poem *Kubla Khan* under the influence of opium but the more strait-laced Wordsworth became infuriated by Coleridge's addiction, and the anti-social behaviour that accompanied it. The two men fell out, and Coleridge spent the following ten years wandering

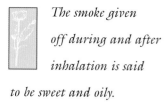

The smoke given off during and after inhalation is said to be sweet and oily.

around Europe, his depressions, illness and opium addiction increasing, and his poetic powers diminished. He moved back to London, living at the house of Dr James Gilman, who temporarily cured him of his addiction but by now it was too late. He died a friendless, opium-addicted alcoholic, unable to bear the depressions.

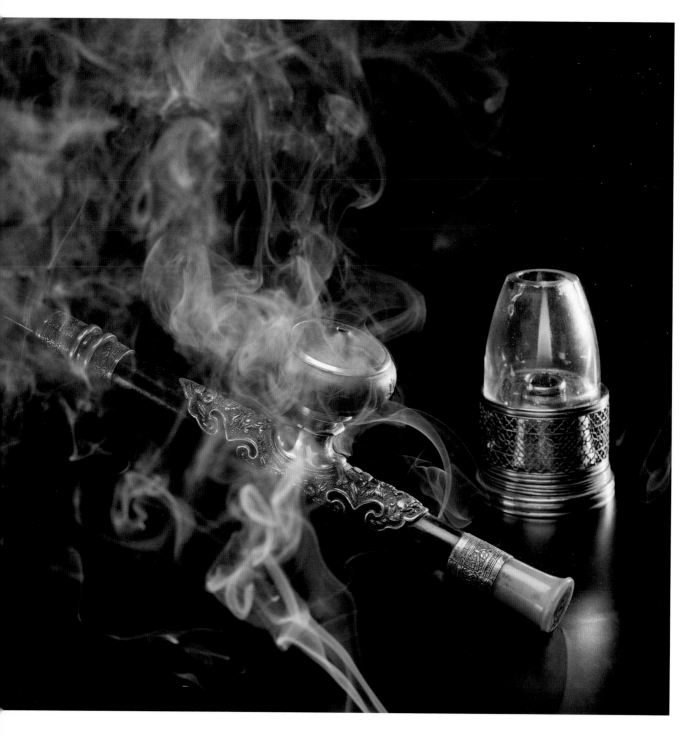

'Here was a panacea … here was the secret of happiness,
about which philosophers had disputed for so many ages,
at once discovered; happiness might now be bought for a
penny, and carried in the waistcoat pocket; portable
ecstasies might be had corked up in a pint bottle; and
peace of mind could be sent down by the mail.'

Thomas de Quincey (1785–1859)

Thomas de Quincey was born in 1785 into a prosperous mercantile family. Aged seventeen, and happily swept away by the romantic notions of the age, de Quincey travelled to Wales, and then lived incognito in London, forming a relationship with a young prostitute, Ann, who would haunt his writings for the rest of his life. In 1803, and reconciled with his family, de Quincey entered Worcester College, Oxford, where he quickly befriended the visiting Coleridge. Like Coleridge, de Quincey had been prescribed laudanum for childhood illness, and together the two students experimented with its hallucinogenic and visionary properties. Whilst at Oxford, de Quincey kept a silver bottle of laudanum at his elbow, steadily increasing his dose. He remained an addict for the rest of his life. In 1803, de Quincey visited the Wordsworths at Grasmere. They were appalled at de Quincey's opium intake, and furthermore, at a relationship de Quincey formed with a local girl Margaret Simpson. Even when the couple married, the Wordsworths remained highly unimpressed and de Quincey was shunted back to London, where he made a bare living writing for the famous periodicals of the time. The family were almost on their knees when de Quincey struck gold in 1821 and published *Confessions of an Opium Eater* in *The London Magazine*. *Confessions* was immediately a best-seller. Ostensibly the book was a journalistic exposé of the moral and physical dangers of opium addiction. After Margaret's death in 1857, de Quincey became even more of recluse and eccentric, locked in his opium dreams until his own death. He did not live long enough to 'enjoy' the discovery of heroin and the hypodermic needle.

'More than fidelity, opium night, I desire the elixir of your lips where love flaunts itself.'

Les Fleurs de Mal by Charles Baudelaire (1821–67)

Baudelaire was a sensual French poet, translator, and literary and art critic. A dissident at school, he quickly abandoned his legal studies to join Delacroix and Daumier, Gautier, Honore de Balzac and Alphonse Karr in Paris' Latin Quarter. These artists established the Club des Haschinchins in the Ile Saint-Louis apartments of painter Fernand Boissard. This was a club for opium and other drug experimentation. It was during this time that Baudelaire, along with a taste for the bohemian high-life, contracted the venereal disease that would eventually kill him. When Baudelaire came into his inheritance in April 1842, he rapidly degenerated into louche extravagance. By 1843, he was regularly smoking opium with his bohemian consorts and writing anguished love poetry to a Mulato woman known as Jeanne Duval. Before long, the debts began to mount. No longer able to afford the vast quantities of opium he had become used to, his life-long bouts of depression began to cripple Baudelaire. In 1857, when his masterpiece *Les Fleurs du Mal* was shredded by the censors for being pornographic, Baudelaire was committed to a nursing home, where he died aged 47.

'At the side of the bed, with a bottle of gin on the rickety table between them, sat two hideous leering, painted monsters, wearing the dress of women. The smell of opium was in the room, as well as the smell of spirits'.

Green Anchor Lane by Wilkie Collins (1824–89)

Wilkie Collins started off life as an unsuccessful lawyer. He happily swapped his wig and gown for a flamboyant literary lifestyle. He devoured mistresses and fine wines, and became the master of the nineteenth century mystery story. He was introduced to opium at the age of nine – Coleridge happened to be a family friend. The broken poet would confide to Collins' mother about his struggle with opium addiction – to which Harriet Collins would reply; 'Mr Coleridge, do not cry; if the opium really does you any good, and you must have it, why do not you go and get it?' At the age of 30 Collins developed agonising neuralgic pains caused by rheumatic gout. Laudanum eased the pain, and Collins quickly became addicted, carrying a silver flask of the preparation everywhere he went. In 1851, he met Charles Dickens. The two

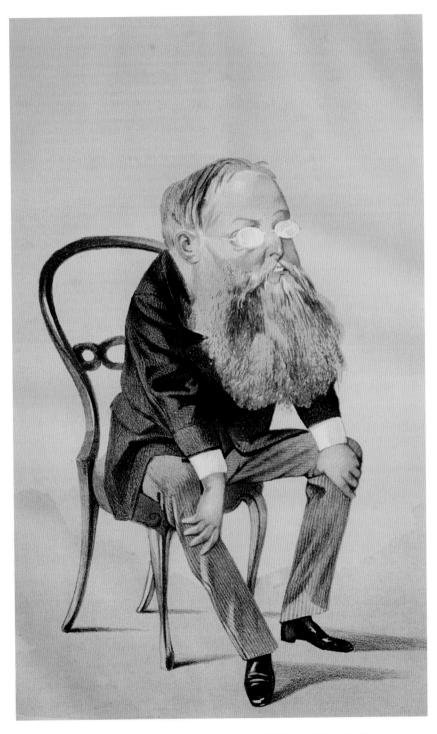

writers collaborated, and Collins published his major work *The Woman in White* in Dickens' periodical *Household Words*, in 1860. By the time he published *The Moonstone* in 1868, Collins' fiction was clouded by opium hallucinations, and by the end of his life, Collins was taking enough opium every day to kill twelve people.

Wilkie Collins.

'Shaking from head to toe, the man whose scattered consciousness has thus fantastically pieced itself together at length rises, supports his trembling frame upon his arms, and looks around. He is in the meanest and closest of small rooms. Through the ragged window curtain, the light of early day steals in from a miserable court. He lies, dressed, across a large unseemly bed, upon a bedstead that has indeed given way under the weight upon it. Lying, also dressed and also across the bed, not longwise, are a Chinaman, a Lascar, and a haggard woman. The first two are in a sleep or stupor; the last is blowing at a kind of pipe to kindle it. And as she blows, and shading it with her lean hand, concentrates its red spark of light, it serves in the dim morning as a lamp to show him what he sees of her.

"Another?" says this woman, in a querulous, rattling whisper. "Have another?"

He looks about him, with his hand to his forehead. "Ye've smoked as many as five since ye come in at midnight," the woman goes on, as she chronically complains. "Poor me, poor me, my head is so bad. Them two come in after ye. Ah, poor me, the business is slack, is slack! Few Chinamen about the Docks, and fewer Lascars, and no ships coming in, these say! Here's another ready for ye, deary. Ye'll remember like a good soul, won't ye, that the market price is dreffle high just now? More nor three shillings and sixpence for a thimbleful! And ye'll remember that nobody but me (and Jack Chinaman t'other side the court; but he can't do it as well as me) has the true secret of mixing it? Ye'll pay up accordingly, deary, won't ye?"

She blows at the pipe as she speaks, and, occasionally
bubbling at it, inhales much of its contents.

"O me, O me, my lungs is weak, my lungs is bad! It's
nearly ready for ye, deary. Ah, poor me, poor me, my poor
hand shakes like to drop off! I see ye coming-to, and I ses
to my poor self, 'I'll have another ready for him, and he'll
bear in mind the market price of opium, and pay according.
O my poor head! I makes my pipes of old penny ink-bottles,
ye see, deary – this is one – and I fits-in a mouthpiece,
this way, and I takes my mixter out of this thimble with
this little horn spoon; and so I fills, deary. Ah, my poor
nerves! I got Heavens-hard drunk for sixteen year afore I
took to this; but this don't hurt me, not to speak of. And it
takes away the hunger as well as wittles, deary."

She hands him the nearly-emptied pipe, and sinks back,
turning over on her face.

He rises unsteadily from the bed, lays the pipe upon the
hearth-stone, draws back, draws back the ragged curtain,
and looks with repugnance at his three companions. He
notices that the woman has opium-smoked herself into a
strange likeness of the Chinaman. His form of cheek, eye,
and temple, and his colour, are repeated in her. Said
Chinaman convulsively wrestles with one of his many Gods
or Devils, perhaps, and snarls horribly. The Lascar laughs
and dribbles at the mouth. The hostess is still.'

**Charles Dickens (1812–70) from his
unfinished novel *The Mystery of Edwin Drood***

The son of a debtor imprisoned in the Marshalsea Prison, Charles Dickens was put to work as a young child in Warren's Blacking Factory. His father was released when he was 12, and Dickens was finally able to attend school. By 15, he was working as an office boy and studying shorthand by night. Quickly he became a court reporter and began to publish stories and sketches under the famous pseudonym 'Boz'. *The Pickwick Papers*, *Oliver Twist* and *Nicholas Nickleby* followed quickly. By 1853, Dickens was an established, acclaimed writer, touring Italy with Wilkie Collins. Dickens suffered terribly from asthma, and Collins suggested opium as a cure – it seemed to work, and he became increasingly dependent on the drug. In 1867, Dickens had a stroke, but against doctor's advice, compulsively carried on working. His last, and unfinished, novel *The Mystery of Edwin Drood* was written on his deathbed, under the influence of opium. It explores London's dark opium underworld and the violent, uneasy fantasies of its inhabitants.

'He knew that for her, he only existed when they smoked.'

Love letter to Louise de Coligny-Châtillon
by Guillaume Apollinaire (1880–1918)

Apollinaire was perhaps one of the most innovative and exuberant avant-garde French poets of the twentieth century. The son of a Polish émigrée and an Italian officer, he kept his origins secret. Left more or less to himself, he went at the age of 20 to Paris, where he led a bohemian life. Several months spent in Germany in 1901 had a profound effect on him and helped to awaken him to his poetic vocation. He fell under the spell of the Rhineland and later recaptured the beauty of its forests and its legends in his poetry. More important, he fell in love with a young Englishwoman, Annie Playden, whom he pursued, unsuccessfully, as far as London; his romantic disappointment inspired him to write his famous *'Chanson du mal-aimé'* ('Song of the Poorly Loved'). After his return to

Paris, Apollinaire became well known as a writer and a habitué of the cafes patronized by literary men. He became friends with Maurice de Vlaminck, André Derain, Raoul Dufy, and Pablo Picasso – with the latter, he collaborated to produce a description of the aesthetics of Cubism, *Peintures cubistes* (1913). With the bohemian Monmartre set, Apollinaire experimented with opium, and published his first volume of poetry, *L'Enchanteur pourrissant* ('The Rotting Magician', 1909), a strange dialogue in poetic prose between the magician Merlin and the nymph Viviane. In 1914, Apollinaire went to Nice, where his opium taking developed into a serious habit. He was besotted with a woman named Louise de Coligny-Châtillon, otherwise known as Lou, who loved him... but only inside the opium den. Outside and sober, she appeared to have more of an aversion to him, and her rejection devastated Apollinaire. Later that year, he enlisted, became a second lieutenant in the infantry, and received a head wound in 1916. Discharged, he returned to Paris and published his significant collection of avante-garde poetry, *Calligrammes* (1918), which was dominated by images of war and his obsession with a new love affair. Weakened by war wounds, he died of Spanish influenza, aged 38.

'There were opium dens where one could buy oblivion, dens of horror where the memory of old sins could be destroyed by the madness of sins that were new'

The Picture of Dorian Gray by Oscar Wilde (1854–1900)

Oscar Wilde was the son of an eminent Dublin surgeon. He was a prodigious child, and won scholarships to both Trinity College, Dublin, and Magdalen College, Oxford, where, as a disciple of Walter Pater he founded the Aesthetic Movement, advocating 'art for art's sake'. Dressed in velvet jackets, knee breeches and black silk stockings, Wilde, along with the artist Aubrey Beardsley, haunted the East London opium dens, playing out the languorous drama of the aesthete dandy. He published stories, and became renowned for his biting, witty, theatrical satires. He loved to drink absinthe, smoke opium-laced cigarettes and indulge himself. However, his decadent lifestyle was stolen away when he was imprisoned in Reading Gaol in 1895, for his alleged homosexual relationship with Lord Alfred Douglas, something which he was never to recover from. In the final decade of his life, Wilde wrote and published nearly all his major works; and in his macabre novel *The Picture of Dorian Gray* he portrays a character Dorian who indulges in 'unspeakable sins'.

'Once a junkie, always a junkie. You can stop using junk, but you are never off the first habit.'

William Burroughs (1914–97)

William Burroughs was born in St Louis, Missouri in 1914. After a series of jobs following university, Burroughs moved to New York in 1943, where he became friends with Jack Kerouac and Allen Ginsberg. Their friendship lead to the whirlwind Beat movement, characterised by experimental, erratic prose, nightmarish, wild and sexually-explicit poetry and journeys into the intoxicated subconscious. Burroughs first took morphine about 1944, and he soon became addicted to heroin. In 1949 he moved with his second wife to Mexico, where in 1951 he accidentally shot and killed her in a drunken prank. Fleeing Mexico, he wandered through the Amazon region of South America, heavily addicted to heroin, desperately depressed and unable to write. He returned to America and checked himself into a rehabilitation clinic. Clean of the opiates and rejuvenated, Burroughs completed his famous books – *Junkie: Confessions of an Unredeemed Drug Addict* and *The Naked Lunch* (1959), satires on the grotesque world of addiction in which the drug user is preyed upon. William Burroughs concluded that all addiction is bad for writing.

'I'm in the mood for a pipe.'

Graham Greene (1904–91)

Greene is the best-loved English writer of this century. His novels, most famously *Brighton Rock* and *The End of the Affair* are on every school syllabus, and have been made into classic films. But Greene's private life was an emotional roller-coaster, often lived on the brink of suicide. After running away from school, Greene was sent to London to a psychoanalyst in whose house he lived while under treatment. He went on to study at Balliol College, Oxford, converted to Roman Catholicism in 1926, and married Vivien Dayrell-Browning the following year. He moved to London and worked for *The Times* as a copy editor, and published his first book of verse, *Babbling April*. After the success of his first novel, *The Man Within* (1929), Greene quit *The Times* and travelled widely for much of the next three decades, working as a freelance journalist, and staying in seedy hotels in Vietnam, Indonesia and the Continent. He liked the idea of being dissolute, and found relief from the boredom of his own existence in alcohol, opium and a

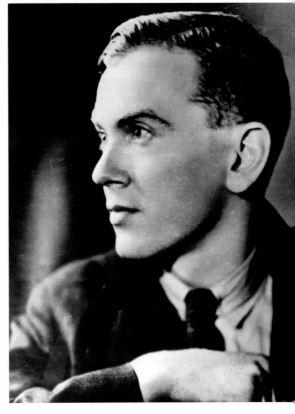

 Graham Greene.

series of relationship with women – long-term lovers, prostitutes and all that falls in-between. This underworld of moral decay and adventure permeates his fiction, which is often characterised by criminals, violence and danger. During the Second World War, Greene worked for the Foreign Office and was stationed for a while at Freetown, Sierra Leone, the scene of another of his best-known novels, *The Heart of the Matter* (1948). He spent the rest of his life between London and the continent, a hugely successful novelist, who liked to live on the brink, and Continued sporadically smoking opium: often after a good lunch he'd say 'I'm in the mood for a pipe'.

'Opium is the least stupid smell in the world.'

Pablo Picasso (1881–1973)

Pablo Picasso was probably the most famous artist of the twentieth century. During his artistic career, which lasted more than 75 years, he created thousands of works, not only paintings but also sculptures, prints and ceramics, using all kinds of materials. He almost single-handedly created modern art. Picasso was born in Malaga, Spain, son of an artist, Jose Ruiz, and Maria Picasso. An artistic prodigy, Picasso, at the age of 14, completed the one-month qualifying examination of the Academy of Fine Arts in Barcelona in one day. From there he went to the Academy of San Fernando in Madrid, returning in 1900 to Barcelona, and then to Paris. This period was known as the 'blue period' because Picasso was so poor that he could not afford to paint in any other colour. During this period, he would spend his days in Paris studying the masterworks at the Louvre and his nights enjoying the company of fellow artists at cabarets like the Lapin Agile. In 1905, there was a radical shift of mood in Picasso's painting – he became interested in circus performers and musicians as subjects, and their colourful shapes and movements began to dominate his paintings. This period was known as the 'rose period'. In 1907, Picasso painted 'Les Demoiselles d'Avignon', considered the watershed picture of the twentieth century. He met Georges Braque, and together they developed and systematised the Cubist movement. The ten years that followed were a period of rich productivity, and the wild, temperamental bohemian living for which Picasso is famous. He began to experiment with opium, alongside Cocteau and Apollinaire but Picasso was an artist driven by criticism, propelled by hard-work and the desire to be successful. While under the influence of opium Picasso found that his imagination and his vision became more acute – but that his desire to paint what he saw diminished seriously. It was this threat of blissful sterility that was opium's most profound influence on the artist, ironically galvanising him into greater production.

> 'Everything one does in life, even love, occurs in an
> express train racing toward death. To smoke opium is to
> get out of the train while it is still moving. It is to
> concern oneself with something other than life or death.'

Jean Cocteau (1889–1963)

This flamboyant French poet, novelist, dramatist, and filmmaker, grew up in the cultivated Parisian pre-1914 bourgeoisie. At 19 he published his first volume of poems, *La Lampe d'Aladin* ('Aladdin's Lamp'). He became fascinated by theatre and ballet, and began to write plays. During war, Cocteau served as an ambulance driver on the Belgian front. Intermittently, he returned to Paris, and entered the bohemian world of modern art then emerging in Montparnasse. There he met painters such as Pablo Picasso and Amadeo Modigliani and writers such as Max Jacob and Guillaume Apollinaire. Opium was a vital feature in this new art scene and he felt that his work when on opium was far more interesting than without. Soon after the war, Max Jacob introduced Cocteau to the beautiful 16-year-old poetic prodigy Raymond Radiguet. The two became lovers, and when Radiguet tragically died in 1923, at the age of 21, Cocteau spiralled into a devastating opium addiction. After a long period in a sanatorium, the rejuvenated Cocteau embarked on his most powerful surrealist works – his films *Le Sang d'un poète* and *La Machine infernale, La belle et la bête* (1945), *Orphée* (1950), and *Les enfants terribles* (1950). Most recently he has been referred to as the Grand Master of Priory of Sion in the book *The Holy Blood and the Holy Grail* (M Baigent, H Lincoln and R Leigh).

As happened in the last few decades of the nineteenth century, the twentieth century also saw its own *fin de siécle* and the rise in the fashion world of 'heroin chic'. Many designers and artists made their models appear emaciated, as if they were 'strung out' on heroin, with dark circles under the eyes. Clothes, make-up and advertising campaigns all reinforced the heroin look. Sadly, some of the models took the image into reality and became heroin addicts themselves, eager to suppress their appetites and have the 'Look'. The supermodel Gia died from an AIDS-related illness which was caught through a shared needle.

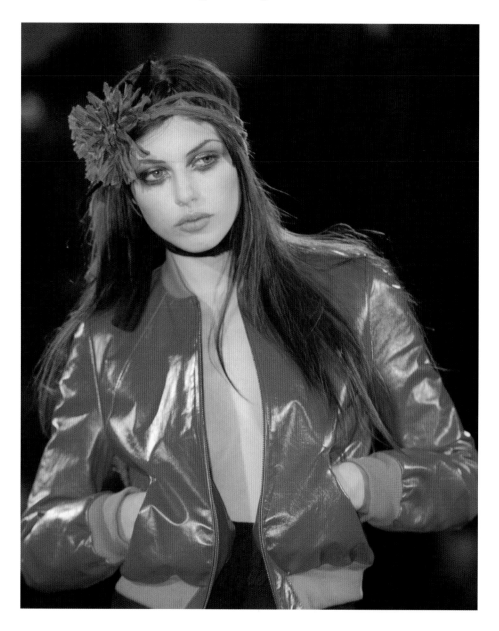

Many designers and artists made their models appear emaciated, as if they were 'strung out' on heroin, with dark circles under the eyes.

From ancient times to now, the opium poppy has featured heavily in spiritual beliefs and within the occult world. For the Sumerians poppies were sacred to their moon goddess, Nin Harsig, and were said to be her flowers of dreaming and a gate into the otherworld. Indeed Culpeper refers to it in his famous *Herbal* as a lunar flower.

In Greek mythology Demeter, the Goddess of Fertility and Harvest, loses her daughter Persephone to Hades, God of the Underworld. Driven to despair she wanders the Earth searching for Persephone and forgets to bring the harvest for a time. It is only in the places that the people treat her hospitably that she brings the barley and wheat to ripen. In the city of Mecone, or City of Poppies, she goes out into the fields and there cuts open the poppy pods and partakes of the latex in order to overcome the pain of losing her daughter. She falls into a state of sleep. Although statues and images of Demeter usually portray her clutching a sheaf of barley there are also some, particularly from Crete, where she is found holding poppies. In the town of Eleusis, Mystery rituals were held in Demeter's honour and again poppies were used to decorate her altars. Opium was taken by the initiates to aid in the forgetting of the sadness of the death of the year, the short drug-induced sleep being a symbol for the passage of winter before the rebirth of the year again in the spring. The twin brothers Thanatos and Hypnos, Greek Gods of Death and Sleep, are represented as carrying or crowned by poppies.

For the Romans, the poppy was a powerful symbol of sleep and death. Somnus, the God of Sleep, is often portrayed as a small boy carrying a bunch of poppies and an opium horn, whilst another popular image for the Romans was that of a figure bending over a woman, pouring poppy juice onto her eyes. The poppy also was part of the mysteries of Ceres, the Roman Goddess of Fertility and counterpart to Demeter; a famous statue shows her holding a torch and poppy pods.

Christianity gave poppy symbolism a new twist; poppies can be found carved into the benches of some medieval churches, representing the belief that we all rest in anticipation of the Day of Judgement although cynics added that it also represented the slumber begun during the priest's sermons.

In the 1800s, during the Occult Revival, many mystics experimented with many kinds of drugs in order to achieve heightened states of consciousness which they linked to the mystic trance.

'The mystical life is the centre of all that I do and all that I think and all that I write.'

William Butler Yeats (1865–1939)

Yeats, the Nobel Prize-winning Irish poet, dramatist, and prose writer, was born at Sandymount, near Dublin, Ireland in 1865. His father and mother were both artists, and Yeats himself studied art for three years, before discovering his talent for writing in his early twenties. He published his first book in 1886 – a little play entitled *Mosada*. This was followed by two collections of poetry, *The Wanderings of Oisin* (1889) and *The Wind Among the Reeds* (1899). Yeats became best known for his unremitting commitment to Irish independence, but in his poetry he cultivated a profound and transcendent mythology based on his explorations into opium and the occult. He joined the Theosophical Society, studied the visionary writings of William Blake, and became interested in a wide range of esoteric sciences, including cheiromancy (palmistry), astrology, chromopathy (healing by colours) and polygraphics (automatic writing). He lectured and wrote on the esoteric, and used opium and other drugs to connect with the deepest and most universal springs of life through the subconscious. In 1890, he joined the famous Hermetic Order of the Golden Dawn, taking the magical motto

'Demon Est Deus Inversus', and was a member of the Rhymer's Club in Paris, consisting of other occultists who were experimenting with drugs to achieve altered states of consciousness, the most famous of whom was Aleister Crowley.

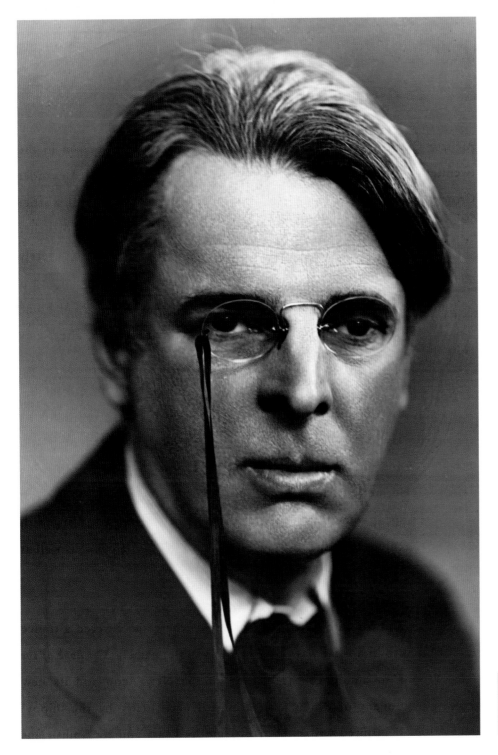

William Butler Yeats.

119

'She it is, she, that found me

In the morphia honeymoon;

With silk and steel she bound me,

In her poisonous milk she drowned me,

Even now her arms surround me,

Stifling me into the swoon'

Thirst by Aleister Crowley (1875–1947)

Aleister Crowley was probably the single most influential person in the twentieth century drug-taking culture. He was born Edward Alexander Crowley on October 12th 1875 in Leamington, Warwickshire into a strict Christian sect called the Plymouth Brethren. His father was a preacher and owner of Crowley's Ales. During his childhood he was so severely mistreated by his family that his health was seriously undermined and it was in these years that Crowley's anti-Christianity was formed. At home the only book he was allowed to read was the Bible. However, after years in different schools he completed his studies in chemistry at King's College, London and then Trinity College, Cambridge. Crowley intended to become a chemist or perhaps enter the diplomatic corps but he never graduated. He became more interested in comparative theology and mountaineering and was in fact a Cambridge Blue in chess. In 1898 he joined the Hermetic Order of the Golden Dawn, a quasi-masonic magical society and spent some years in Paris where he began experimenting with opium, laudanum, hashish, cocaine, mescaline and ethyl-alcohol as well as ritual magick, a potent brew for anyone.

In 1904 he and his wife Rose went to Egypt where she entered a trance and dictated to him what was to become his Bible, namely *The Book of the Law*, a book to announce the coming of the New Aeon and its new philosophies, many of which were espoused particularly by the 'hippy' generation. It inspired writers such as Timothy Leary and rock musicians such as Jimmy Page of the rock band Led Zeppelin. In 1921 he wrote *Diary of a Drug Fiend* which was immediately seized by His Majesty's Customs. The book traces the story of a young, well-to-do couple's fall into drug addiction and their subsequent cure and, contrary to media opinion of the time, is by no means pro-drugs. His writings and diaries are riddled with references to drug-taking and his treatise on Hashish in his magazine *The Equinox* is seminal. He took heroin for the first time in 1919 for asthma, an illness which had affected him from childhood, and used it until his death in 1947, aged 72 when his doctor withdrew his prescription.

'I had become a bounden slave in the travels of opium,
And my labours and my orders had taken a colouring from
my dreams'

Ligeia by Edgar Allen Poe (1809–49)

Edgar Allan Poe was born in Boston in 1809, the son of itinerant actors. His mother died when he was 11, and the young poet was put into the care of a family friend. Their relationship was always strained, and when Poe dropped out of the University of Virginia, his guardian refused to support him. Poe went to Boston to write poetry. Financial hardship forced him to join the army – but his guardian came to the rescue and bought him out. Poe went to New York City and then to Philadelphia, where he became interested in the occult. He began drinking heavily, womanising, and taking opium to dull his agonising bouts of paranoia and penetrating depression. At this time, he began to publish the feverish, supernatural and grotesque short stories for which he is famous, including *The Fall of the House of Usher*. In 1836, he married his 13-year-old cousin Virginia Clemm. When Clemm died tragically young in 1846, Poe became horrendously depressed, and journeyed to the depths of opium addiction and alcoholism. It was to Virginia that he wrote what was to be his favourite poem, *Ligeia*. He was desperate to re-marry, and began to proposition an older, beautiful clairvoyant widow, Mrs Shelton. Initially, she thought his protestations no more than poetic games; when she realised the desperation of his passion, she agreed to marry him on the condition that he never drank again. Of course, Poe promised – but he never managed to keep dry. What is more, Mrs Shelton's mother disapproved of the match and circulated rumours that Poe had been unfaithful. Mrs Shelton confronted Poe, and their argument was acrimonious. Devastated, Poe left her house and went to the chemist to buy 3 grams of opium. Then, on the train to Boston, he swallowed the lot. It was only the intervention of the friend who collected him at Boston that saved his life. He died a few months later, possibly through contracting rabies, collapsing in a Baltimore tavern, and was buried next to his wife.

'There are far worse things awaiting man than death.'

Bela Lugosi (1882–1956)

Bela Lugosi was born in Hungary in 1882. Aged 11 he ran away from home, and began working in odd jobs, including stage acting. He studied at the Budapest Academy of Theatrical Arts and made his stage debut in 1901. From 1913 to 1919 he was a member of the National Theatre. Lugosi left to go to Germany in 1919, and in 1921, emigrated to the United States. It was a dangerous move – Lugosi spoke hardly any English and his chances of working in the academy theatres were extremely slim. He hardly worked at all, until he was picked to play the title role in a Broadway production of Bram Stoker's novel *Dracula*. The production was a huge success and ran for three years. Soon after, Universal Pictures made a film adaptation in 1931. With his slow, thickly-accented voice and handsome, brooding looks, Lugosi was the obvious choice to play the Count. The film catapulted Lugosi to fame, and he was recognised as something of a ladies man. A string of horror movies followed *Dracula*, many of which had been penned by Edgar Allen Poe – *Murders in the Rue Morgue* (1932), *White Zombie* (1932), *Island of Lost Souls* (1933), *The Black Cat* (1934) and *The Raven* (1935). By now, he was hopelessly typecast in a genre that had become unpopular. Ten years later Lugosi had declined into poverty, obscurity, and a growing dependence on morphine, a shadow of his former self. He would constantly inject himself with morphine and try to sleep away his painful memories. In 1955 he voluntarily committed himself to the state hospital in Norwalk,

Bela Lugosi.

California, as a drug addict. He was released later that year and began to depend on a friendship with Ed Wood, Jr., the man regarded by many as the most comprehensively inept director in film history. Lugosi starred in such unintentionally cult classics as *Bride of the Monster* and *Plan 9 from Outer Space*, but his health remained poor. After being hospitalised again for morphine addiction he died on August 16th 1956. He was buried, as he wished, wearing the long black cape that he had worn in *Dracula*. His deterioration was immortalised in the film *Ed Wood* directed by Tim Burton in which Martin Landau won an Oscar for his role as Bela Lugosi.

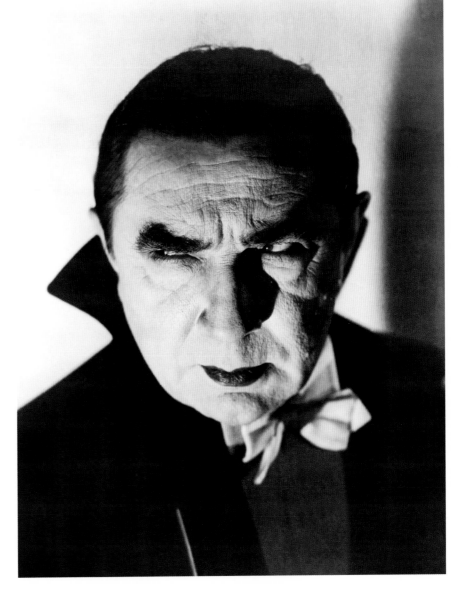

The illicit drug trade touches millions of lives, in both the developed and the developing world. Its most negative impact is among the vulnerable and marginalised within our society. The UN estimates that over 180 million people worldwide are consuming drugs, 13 million of which are abusing opiates and 9 million of whom are addicted to heroin. Economic reliance on the drug trade leaves many individuals open to exploitation by criminal organisations. This threatens the health of all ages and ultimately the health of the global community. However, for the first time in recent history, global production of opium is no longer growing but is showing signs of stabilising and even a decline. Illicit opium production declined at the onset of the Millennium by at least 17% and that was 15% lower than 1994. The production of opium is concentrated in an ever-dwindling number of countries, which makes efforts of alternative development an increasingly viable option in order to achieve the targets which were set out in the 1998 UN Assembly. These targets aim at a substantial reduction and elimination of opium production by the year 2008. Whether these targets will be met remains to be seen as history has shown time and again that opium is too precious a commodity for the corrupt parts of society to relinquish.

We end this story of opium where we began, with a few lines on morphine from the master drug fiend himself.

'And you, you puritan others
 who have missed the morphia craving,
cry scorn if I call you brothers,
Curl lip at my manic ravings,
Fools, seven times beguiled,
You have not known her? Well!
There was never a need she smiled
To harry you into hell!'

***Diary of a Drug Fiend* by Aleister Crowley
(1875–1947)**

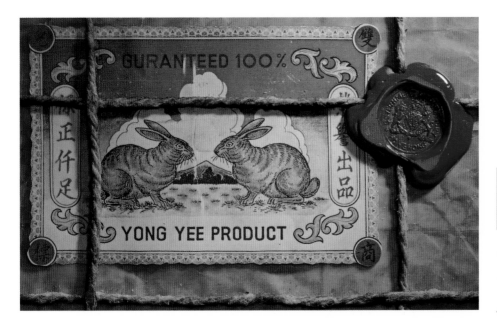

The Yong Yee label – a popular brand of opium traded in South China – with the red wax seal of the official government chemist.

INDEX